Plant Based Diet

Recipes

50+ Easy Recipes Ready in under 30
Minutes

Margaret Hooper

TABLE OF CONTENTS

INTRODUCTION

A plant-based diet emphasizes the use of whole plant foods. This means eliminating all high-refined foods such as oil, refined sugar, and bleached flour. In addition to eliminating these foods, you will begin to reduce or eliminate your consumption of egg, dairy products, and meat! Whole grains, tomatoes, fruits, tubers, and all varieties of legumes will be available instead.

Giving yourself a variety in your diet is the secret to a healthy plant-based diet. Leafy greens will be relevant, but they will not provide enough calories on their own! When you think about it, you'd have to eat a lot of kale to meet your calorie targets. Calories are vital because you will feel deprived and drained if you don't consume enough of them. As a result, the plant-based diet is chock-full of delectable foods for you to sample!

veggies and Fruits are often rich in fiber and carbs. Moreover, they have high water content, unlike most unhealthy snacks you eat that tend to have low water content or are low in fiber. Without fiber and water content, the digestive system can process the food quickly, which often leaves your stomach empty, causing you to overeat. Fruits and veggies make you feel full for longer as it takes longer for the digestive system to process them, thereby limiting the amount of food you eat.

Because of this, people whose diet is comprised mainly of fruits and vegetables are likely to have a lower body mass index and are less susceptible to obesity, diabetes, and heart disease. There was a study back in 2018 conducted to gauge the effectiveness of a plant-based diet for treating obesity. Here, the researcher observed 75 participants who were obese. Some were selected to go on a plant-based diet, whereas others were told to continue to eat as they were.

To no one's surprise, four months later, the vegan group showed a tremendous loss in weight. On average, they lost about 14.33 pounds (6.5 kilograms). Most of this weight loss is the loss of fat mass. Moreover, subjects reported having better insulin sensitivity. All of these changes were not found in the group that followed their usual diet, which consisted of meat.

An extensive study was conducted in 2009, spanning more than 60,000 people. It found that vegans tend to have the lowest average BMI than lacto-ovo vegetarians (who eat dairy and eggs), then pescatarians (who eat fish but no meat).

BREAKFAST RECIPES

1. Chickpea Flour Frittata

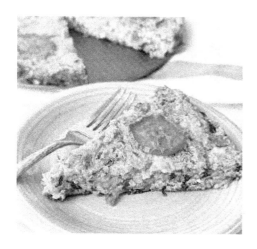

Preparation time: 10 minutes

Cooking time: 50 minutes

Servings: 6

Ingredients:

- 1 medium green bell pepper, cored, chopped
- 1 cup chopped greens
- 1 cup cauliflower florets, chopped
- ½ cup chopped broccoli florets
- ½ of a medium red onion, peeled, chopped
- ¼ teaspoon salt
- ½ cup chopped zucchini

For the Batter:

- ¼ cup cashew cream
- 1 ½ cup chickpea flour
- ½ cup chopped cilantro
- ½ teaspoon salt
- ¼ teaspoon cayenne pepper
- ½ teaspoon dried dill
- ¼ teaspoon ground black pepper
- ¼ teaspoon dried thyme
- ½ teaspoon ground turmeric
- 1 tablespoon olive oil
- 1 ½ cup water

Directions:

1. Switch on the oven, then set it to 375 degrees F and let it preheat. Take a 9-inch pie pan, grease it with oil, and then set aside until required.
2. Put all the vegetables in your large bowl, sprinkle with salt and then toss until combined.
3. Prepare the batter by adding all of its ingredients except for thyme, dill, and cilantro, and then pulse until combined and smooth.
4. Pour the batter over the vegetables, add dill, thyme, and cilantro, and then stir until combined.
5. Put the batter into your prepared pan, spread evenly, and then bake for 45 to 50 minutes until done and inserted toothpick into frittata comes out clean.
6. When done, let the frittata rest for 10 minutes, cut it into slices, and then serve.

Nutrition: Calories: 153 Fat: 4 g Protein: 7 g Carbs: 20 g

2. <u>Potato Pancakes</u>

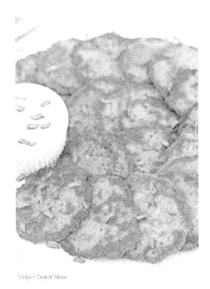

Preparation time: 10 minutes

Cooking time: 20 minutes

Servings: 10

Ingredients:

- ½ cup white whole-wheat flour
- 3 large potatoes, grated
- ½ of a medium white onion, peeled, grated
- 1 jalapeno, minced
- 2 green onions, chopped
- 1 tablespoon minced garlic
- 1 teaspoon salt
- ¼ teaspoon baking powder
- ¼ teaspoon ground pepper
- 4 tablespoons olive oil

Directions:

1. Take a large bowl, place all the ingredients except for oil and then stir until well combined; stir in 1 to 2 tablespoons water if needed to mix the batter.
2. Take a large skillet pan, place it over medium-high heat, add 2 tablespoons of oil and then let it heat.
3. Scoop the pancake mixture in portions into the pan, shape each portion like a pancake and then cook for 5 to 7 minutes per side until pancakes turn golden brown and thoroughly cooked.
4. When done, transfer the pancakes to a plate, add more oil into the pan and then cook more pancakes in the same manner. Serve straight away.

Nutrition: Calories: 69 Fat: 1 g Protein: 2 g Carbs: 12 g

3. Chocolate Chip Pancakes

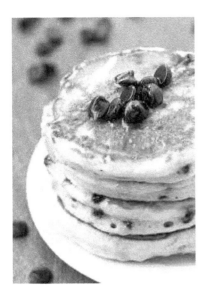

Preparation time: 5 minutes

Cooking time: 10 minutes

Servings: 6

Ingredients:

- 1 cup white whole-wheat flour
- ½ cup chocolate chips, vegan, unsweetened
- 1 tablespoon baking powder
- ¼ teaspoon salt
- 2 teaspoons coconut sugar
- 1 ½ teaspoon vanilla extract, unsweetened
- 1 cup almond milk, unsweetened
- 2 tablespoons coconut butter, melted
- 2 tablespoons olive oil

Directions:

1. Take a large bowl, place all the ingredients except for oil and chocolate chips, and then stir until well combined. Add chocolate chips, and then fold until just mixed.
2. Take a large skillet pan, place it over medium-high heat, add 1 tablespoon oil and then let it heat.
3. Scoop the pancake mixture in portions into the pan, shape each portion like a pancake and then cook for 5 to 7 minutes per side until pancakes turn golden brown and thoroughly cooked.
4. When done, transfer the pancakes to a plate, add more oil into the pan and then cook more pancakes in the same manner. Serve straight away.

Nutrition: Calories: 172 Fat: 6 g Protein: 2.5 g Carbs: 28 g

4. <u>Turmeric Steel-Cut Oats</u>

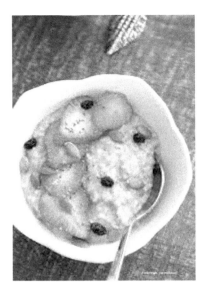

Preparation time: 5 minutes

Cooking time: 10 minutes

Servings: 2

Ingredients:

- ½ cup steel-cut oats
- 1/8 teaspoon salt
- 2 tablespoons maple syrup
- ½ teaspoon ground cinnamon
- 1/3 teaspoon turmeric powder
- ¼ teaspoon ground cardamom
- ¼ teaspoon olive oil
- 1 ½ cups water
- 1 cup almond milk, unsweetened

For the Topping:

- 2 tablespoons pumpkin seeds
- 2 tablespoons chia seeds

Directions:

1. Take a medium saucepan, place it over medium heat, add oats, and then cook for 2 minutes until toasted. Pour in the milk plus water, stir until mixed, and then bring the oats to a boil.
2. Then switch heat to medium-low level, simmer the oats for 10 minutes, and add salt, maple syrup, and spices.
3. Stir until combined, cook the oats for 7 minutes or more until cooked to the desired level and when done, let the oats rest for 15 minutes.
4. When done, divide oats evenly between two bowls, top with pumpkin seeds and chia seeds and then serve.

Nutrition: Calories: 234 Fat: 4 g Protein: 7 g Carbs: 41 g

5. Vegetable Pancakes

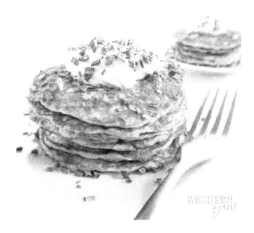

Preparation time: 10 minutes

Cooking time: 20 minutes

Servings: 10

Ingredients:

- 1/3 cup cooked & mashed sweet potato
- 2 cups grated carrots
- 1 cup chopped coriander
- 1 cup cooked spinach
- 3 1/2 ounces chickpea flour
- ½ teaspoon baking powder
- 1 ½ teaspoon salt
- 1 teaspoon ground turmeric
- 2 tablespoons olive oil
- ¾ cup of water

Directions:

1. Take a large bowl, place chickpea flour in it, add turmeric powder, baking powder, and salt, and then stir until combined.
2. Whisk in the water until combined, stir in sweet potatoes until well mixed and then add carrots, spinach, and coriander until well combined.
3. Take a large skillet pan, place it over medium-high heat, add 1 tablespoon oil and then let it heat.
4. Scoop the pancake mixture in portions into the pan, shape each portion like a pancake and then cook for 3 to 5 minutes per side until pancakes turn golden brown and thoroughly cooked.
5. When done, transfer the pancakes to a plate, add more oil into the pan and then cook more pancakes in the same manner. Serve straight away.

Nutrition: Calories: 74 Fat: 0.3 g Protein: 3 g Carbs: 16 g

6. Banana and Chia Pudding

Preparation time: 25 minutes

Cooking time: 12 minutes

Servings: 2

Ingredients:

For the Pudding:

- 2 bananas, peeled
- 4 tablespoons chia seeds
- 2 tablespoons coconut sugar
- ½ teaspoon pumpkin pie spice
- 1/8 teaspoon sea salt
- 1 ½ cup almond milk, unsweetened

For the Bananas:

- 2 bananas, peeled, sliced
- 2 tablespoons coconut flakes
- 1/8 teaspoon ground cinnamon
- 2 tablespoons coconut sugar
- ¼ cup chopped walnuts
- 2 tablespoons almond milk, unsweetened

Directions:

1. Prepare the pudding, place all of its ingredients in a blender except for chia seeds and then pulse until smooth.

2. Pour the batter into a medium saucepan, place it over medium heat, bring the mixture to a boil and then remove the pan from heat.
3. Add chia seeds into the hot banana mixture, stir until mixed, and then let it sit for 5 minutes. Whisk the pudding and then let it chill for 15 minutes in the refrigerator.
4. Meanwhile, prepare the caramelized bananas, take a medium skillet pan, and place it over medium heat.
5. Add banana slices, sprinkle with salt, sugar, and nutmeg, drizzle with milk and then cook for 5 minutes until the mixture has thickened.
6. Assemble the pudding and for this, divide the pudding evenly between two bowls, top with banana slices, sprinkle with walnuts, and then serve.

Nutrition: Calories: 495 Fat: 21 g Protein: 9 g Carbs: 76 g

7. Pumpkin Spice Oatmeal

Preparation time: 5 minutes

Cooking time: 8 minutes

Servings: 2

Ingredients:

- ¼ cup Medjool dates, pitted, chopped
- 2/3 cup rolled oats
- 1 tablespoon maple syrup
- ½ teaspoon pumpkin pie spice
- ½ teaspoon vanilla extract, unsweetened
- 1/3 cup pumpkin puree
- 2 tablespoons chopped pecans
- 1 cup almond milk, unsweetened

Directions:

1. Take a medium pot, place it over medium heat, and then add all the ingredients except for pecans and maple syrup.
2. Stir all the ingredients until combined, and then cook for 5 minutes until the oatmeal has absorbed all the liquid and thickened.
3. When done, divide oatmeal evenly between two bowls, top with pecans, drizzle with maple syrup and then serve.

Nutrition: Calories: 175 Fat: 3.2 g Protein: 5.8 g Carbs: 33 g

8. Peanut Butter Bites

Preparation time: 15 minutes

Cooking time: 0 minutes

Servings: 20 balls

Ingredients:

- 1 cup rolled oats
- 12 Medjool dates, pitted
- ½ cup peanut butter, sugar-free

Directions:

1. Plug in a blender or a food processor, add all the ingredients in its jar, and then cover with the lid. Pulse for 5 minutes until well combined, and then tip the mixture into a shallow dish.
2. Shape the mixture into 20 balls, 1 tablespoon of mixture per ball, and then serve.

Nutrition: Calories: 103.1 Fat: 4.3 g Protein: 2.3 g Carbs: 15.4 g

9. Maple and Cinnamon Overnight Oats

Preparation time: 2 hours & 15 minutes

Cooking time: 0 minutes

Servings: 4

Ingredients:

- 2 cups rolled oats
- ¼ cup chopped pecans
- ¾ teaspoon ground cinnamon
- 1 teaspoon vanilla extract, unsweetened
- 3 tablespoons coconut sugar
- 3 tablespoons maple syrup
- 2 cups almond milk, unsweetened

Directions:

1. Take four mason jars, and then add ½ cup oats, ¼ teaspoon vanilla, and ½ cup milk.
2. Take a small bowl, add maple syrup, cinnamon, and sugar, stir until mixed, add this mixture into the oats mixture and then stir until combined.

3. Cover the jars with the lid and then let them rest in the refrigerator for a minimum of 2 hours or more until thickened.

4. When ready to eat, top the oats with pecans, sprinkle with cinnamon, drizzle with maple syrup and then serve.

Nutrition: Calories: 292 Fat: 9 g Protein: 7 g Carbs: 48 g

10. Beans on Toast

Preparation time: 5 minutes

Cooking time: 10 minutes

Servings: 4

Ingredients:

- 2 cups cooked navy beans
- 1/3 cup sun-dried tomatoes, chopped
- ½ of a medium white onion, peeled, chopped
- 1 teaspoon minced garlic
- 1 tablespoon molasses
- 2 teaspoons soy sauce
- ¼ cup tomato paste
- ¼ cup ketchup
- ¼ teaspoon liquid smoke
- 1 tablespoon olive oil
- ¼ cup of water
- 4 slices of whole-wheat bread

Directions:

1. Take a large skillet pan, place it over medium-high heat, add oil and then let it heat. Add onion, stir in garlic and then cook for 5 minutes until onion begins to brown.
2. Add remaining ingredients except for bread slices, stir until combined, and then cook the mixture for 5

minutes or more until thoroughly hot. Spread the bean batter over the bread slices and then serve.

Nutrition: Calories: 290 Fat: 6 g Protein: 9 g Carbs: 51 g

LUNCH

11. Eggplant and Olives Stew

Preparation time: 10 minutes

Cooking time: 30 minutes

Servings: 4

Ingredients:

- 2 scallions, chopped
- 2 tablespoons avocado oil
- 2 garlic cloves, chopped
- 1 bunch parsley, chopped
- Salt and black pepper to the taste
- 1 teaspoon basil, dried
- 1 teaspoon cumin, dried
- 2 eggplants, roughly cubed
- 1 cup green olives, pitted and sliced
- 3 tablespoons balsamic vinegar
- ½ Cup tomato passata

Directions:

1. Warm-up your pot with the oil on medium heat, put the scallions, garlic, basil, cumin, and sauté for 5 minutes.

2. Add the eggplants and the other ingredients, toss, cook over medium heat for 25 minutes more, divide into bowls and serve.

Nutrition: Calories 93 Fat 1.8g Carbs 18.6g Protein 3.4g

12. Cauliflower and Artichokes Soup

Preparation time: 10 minutes

Cooking time: 25 minutes

Servings: 4

Ingredients:

- 1 pound cauliflower florets
- 1 cup canned artichoke hearts, drained & chopped
- 2 scallions, chopped
- 2 tablespoons olive oil
- 2 garlic cloves, minced
- 6 cups vegetable stock
- Salt and black pepper to the taste
- 2/3 cup coconut cream
- 2 tablespoons cilantro, chopped

Directions:

1. Heat-up a pot with the oil over medium heat, add the scallions and the garlic, and sauté for 5 minutes.
2. Add the cauliflower and the other fixings, toss, bring to a simmer and cook over medium heat for 20 minutes more. Blend the soup using an immersion blender, divide it into bowls and serve.

Nutrition: Calories 207 Fat 17.2g Carbs 14.1g Protein 4.7g

13. Hot Cabbage Soup

Preparation time: 10 minutes

Cooking time: 30 minutes

Servings: 4

Ingredients:

- 3 spring onions, chopped
- 1 green cabbage head, shredded
- 2 tablespoons olive oil
- 1 tablespoon ginger, grated
- 1 teaspoon cumin, ground
- 6 cups vegetable stock
- Salt and black pepper to the taste
- 1 teaspoon hot paprika
- 1 teaspoon chili powder
- 1 tablespoon cilantro, chopped

Directions:

1. Heat-up your pot with the oil over medium heat, add the spring onions, ginger, and the cumin, and sauté for 5 minutes.
2. Add the cabbage and the other ingredients, stir, bring to a simmer and cook over medium heat for 25 minutes more. Ladle the soup into bowls and serve for lunch.

Nutrition: Calories 117 Fat 7.5g Carbs 12.7g Protein 2.8g

14. Classic Black Beans Chili

Preparation time: 10 minutes

Cooking time: 3 hours

Servings: 4

Ingredients:

- ½ cup quinoa
- 2 and ½ cups veggie stock
- 14 ounces canned tomatoes, chopped
- 15 ounces canned black beans, drained
- ¼ cup green bell pepper, chopped
- ¼ cup red bell pepper, chopped
- A pinch of salt and black pepper
- 2 garlic cloves, minced
- 1 carrot, shredded
- 1 small chili pepper, chopped
- 2 teaspoons chili powder
- 1 teaspoon cumin, ground
- A pinch of cayenne pepper
- ½ cup of corn
- 1 teaspoon oregano, dried

For the vegan sour cream:

- A drizzle of apple cider vinegar
- 4 tablespoons water
- ½ cup cashews, soaked overnight and drained
- 1 teaspoon lime juice

Directions:

1. Put the stock in your slow cooker. Add quinoa, tomatoes, beans, red and green bell pepper, garlic, carrot, salt, pepper, corn, cumin, cayenne, chili powder, chili pepper oregano, stir, cover, and cook on high for 3 hours.
2. Meanwhile, put the cashews in your blender. Add water, vinegar, and lime juice and pulse well. Divide beans chili into bowls, top with vegan sour cream, and serve.

Nutrition: Calories 300 Fat 4g Carbs 10g Protein 7g

15. Amazing Potato Dish

Preparation time: 10 minutes

Cooking time: 3 hours

Servings: 4

Ingredients:

- 1 and ½ pounds potatoes, peeled and roughly chopped
- 1 tablespoon olive oil
- 3 tablespoons water
- 1 small yellow onion, chopped
- ½ cup veggie stock cube, crumbled
- ½ teaspoon coriander, ground
- ½ teaspoon cumin, ground
- ½ teaspoon garam masala
- ½ teaspoon chili powder
- Black pepper to the taste
- ½ pound spinach, roughly torn

Directions:

1. Put the potatoes in your slow cooker. Add oil, water, onion, stock cube, coriander, cumin, garam masala, chili powder, black pepper, and spinach.
2. Stir, cover, and cook on high within 3 hours. Divide into bowls and serve. Enjoy!

Nutrition: Calories 270 Fat 4g Carbs 8g Protein 12g

16. Sweet Potatoes and Lentils Delight

Preparation time: 10 minutes

Cooking time: 4 hours and 30 minutes

Servings: 6

Ingredients:

- 6 cups sweet potatoes, peeled and cubed
- 2 teaspoons coriander, ground
- 2 teaspoons chili powder
- 1 yellow onion, chopped
- 3 cups veggie stock
- 4 garlic cloves, minced
- A pinch of sea salt
- black pepper
- 10 ounces canned coconut milk
- 1 cup of water
- 1 and ½ cups red lentils

Directions:

1. Put sweet potatoes in your slow cooker. Add coriander, chili powder, onion, stock, garlic, salt, and pepper, stir, cover and cook on high for 3 hours.
2. Add lentils, stir, cover, and cook for 1 hour and 30 minutes. Add water and coconut milk, stir well, divide into bowls, and serve right away. Enjoy!

Nutrition Calories 300 Fat 10g Carbs 16g Protein 10g

17. Mushroom Stew

Preparation time: 10 minutes

Cooking time: 8 hours

Servings: 4

Ingredients:

- 2 garlic cloves, minced
- 1 celery stalk, chopped
- 1 yellow onion, chopped
- 1 and ½ cups firm tofu, pressed and cubed
- 1 cup of water
- 10 ounces mushrooms, chopped
- 1 pound mixed peas, corn, and carrots
- 2 and ½ cups veggie stock
- 1 teaspoon thyme, dried
- 2 tablespoons coconut flour
- A pinch of sea salt
- Black pepper to the taste

Directions:

1. Put the water and stock in your slow cooker. Add garlic, onion, celery, mushrooms, mixed veggies, tofu, thyme, salt, pepper, and flour.
2. Stir everything, cover, and cook on low for 8 hours. Divide into bowls and serve hot. Enjoy!

Nutrition: Calories 230 Fat 4g Carbs 10g Protein 7g

18. Simple Tofu Dish

Preparation time: 10 minutes

Cooking time: 3 hours

Servings: 6

Ingredients:

- 1 big tofu package, cubed
- 1 tablespoon sesame oil
- ¼ cup pineapple, cubed
- 1 tablespoon olive oil
- 2 garlic cloves, minced
- 1 tablespoon brown rice vinegar
- 2 teaspoon ginger, grated
- ¼ cup soy sauce
- 5 big zucchinis, cubed
- ¼ cup sesame seeds

Directions:

1. In your food processor, mix sesame oil with pineapple, olive oil, garlic, ginger, soy sauce, and vinegar and whisk well.
2. Add this to your slow cooker and mix with tofu cubes. Cover and cook on High within 2 hours and 45 minutes.
3. Add sesame seeds and zucchinis, stir gently, cover, and cook on High for 15 minutes. Divide between plates and serve. Enjoy!

Nutrition: Calories 200 Fat 3g Carbs 9g Protein 10g

19. Special Jambalaya

Preparation time: 10 minutes

Cooking time: 6 hours

Servings: 4

Ingredients:

- 6 ounces soy chorizo, chopped
- 1 and ½ cups celery ribs, chopped
- 1 cup okra
- 1 green bell pepper, chopped
- 16 ounces canned tomatoes and green chilies, chopped
- 2 garlic cloves, minced
- ½ teaspoon paprika
- 1 and ½ cups veggie stock
- a pinch of cayenne pepper
- black pepper to the taste
- a pinch of salt
- 3 cups already cooked wild rice for serving

Directions:

1. Warm-up a pan over medium-high heat, put soy chorizo, stir, brown for a few minutes and transfer to your slow cooker.
2. Also, add celery, bell pepper, okra, tomatoes and chilies, garlic, paprika, salt, pepper, and cayenne to your slow cooker.

3. Stir everything, add the veggie stock, cover the slow cooker, and cook on low for 6 hours. Divide rice between plates, top each serving with your vegan jambalaya and serve hot. Enjoy!

Nutrition: Calories 150 Fat 3g Carbs 15g Protein 9g

20. Chinese Tofu and Veggies

Preparation time: 10 minutes

Cooking time: 4 hours

Servings: 4

Ingredients:

- 14 ounces extra-firm tofu, pressed & cut into medium triangles
- cooking spray
- 2 teaspoons ginger, grated
- 1 yellow onion, chopped
- 3 garlic cloves, minced
- 8 ounces tomato sauce
- ¼ cup hoisin sauce
- ¼ teaspoon coconut aminos
- 2 tablespoons of rice wine vinegar
- 1 tablespoon soy sauce
- 1 tablespoon spicy mustard
- ¼ teaspoon red pepper, crushed
- 2 teaspoons molasses
- 2 tablespoons water
- a pinch of black pepper
- 3 broccoli stalks
- 1 green bell pepper, cut into squares
- 2 zucchinis, cubed

Directions:

1. Warm-up a pan over medium-high heat, add tofu pieces, brown them for a few minutes and transfer to your slow cooker.
2. Heat the pan again over medium-high heat, add ginger, onion, garlic, and tomato sauce, stir, sauté for a few minutes and transfer to your slow cooker as well.
3. Add hoisin sauce, aminos, vinegar, soy sauce, mustard, red pepper, molasses, water, and black pepper, stir gently, cover, and cook on high for 3 hours.
4. Add zucchinis, bell pepper, and broccoli, cover, and cook on high for 1 more hour. Divide between plates and serve right away.

Nutrition: Calories 300 Fat 4g Carbs 14g Protein 13g

DINNER

21. Spicy Grilled Tofu Steak

Preparation time: 15 minutes

Cooking time: 8 minutes

Servings: 4

Ingredients:

1 tbsp. of the following:

- chopped scallion
- chopped cilantro
- soy sauce
- hoisin sauce
- 2 tbsp. oil

¼ tsp of the following:

- salt
- garlic powder
- red chili pepper powder
- ground Sichuan peppercorn powder
- ½ tsp cumin
- 1 pound firm tofu

Directions:

1. Put the tofu on a plate and drain the excess liquid for about 10 minutes. Slice drained tofu into ¾ thick stakes.

2. Stir the cumin, Sichuan peppercorn, chili powder, garlic powder, and salt in a mixing bowl until well-incorporated.
3. In another little bowl, combine soy sauce, hoisin, and 1 teaspoon of oil. Heat a skillet to medium temperature with oil, then carefully place the tofu in the skillet.
4. Sprinkle the spices over the tofu, distributing equally across all steaks. Cook for 3-5 minutes, flip, and put spice on the other side. Cook for an additional 3 minutes.
5. Brush with sauce and plate. Sprinkle some scallion and cilantro and enjoy.

Nutrition: Calories: 155 Carbohydrates: 7.6 g Proteins: 9.9 g Fats: 11.8 g

22. Piquillo Salsa Verde Steak

Preparation time: 15 minutes

Cooking time: 5 minutes

Servings: 8

Ingredients:

- 4 – ½ inch thick slices of ciabatta
- 18 oz. firm tofu, drained
- 5 tbsp. olive oil, extra virgin
- Pinch of cayenne
- ½ t. cumin, ground
- 1 ½ tbsp. sherry vinegar
- 1 shallot, diced
- 8 piquillo peppers (can be from a jar) – drained and cut to ½ inch strips

3 tbsp. of the following:

- parsley, finely chopped
- capers, drained and chopped

Directions:

1. Place the tofu on a plate to drain the excess liquid, and then slice into 8 rectangle pieces. You can either prepare your grill or use a grill pan. If using a grill pan, preheat the grill pan.
2. Mix 3 tablespoons of olive oil, cayenne, cumin, vinegar, shallot, parsley, capers, and piquillo peppers in a

medium bowl to make our salsa Verde. Season to preference with salt and pepper.

3. Using a paper towel, dry the tofu slices. Brush olive oil on each side, seasoning with salt and pepper lightly.
4. Place the bread on the grill and toast for about 2 minutes using medium-high heat. Next, grill the tofu, cooking each side for about 3 minutes or until the tofu is heated through.
5. Place the toasted bread on the plate then the tofu on top of the bread. Gently spoon out the salsa Verde over the tofu and serve.

Nutrition: Calories: 427 Carbohydrates: 67.5 g Proteins: 14.2 g Fats: 14.6 g

23. **Butternut Squash Steak**

Preparation time: 15 minutes

Cooking time: 20 minutes

Servings: 4

Ingredients:

- 2 tbsp. coconut yogurt
- ½ tsp sweet paprika
- 1 ¼ cup low-sodium vegetable broth
- 1 sprig thyme
- 1 finely chopped garlic clove
- 1 big thinly sliced shallot
- 1 tbsp. margarine
- 2 tbsp. olive oil, extra virgin
- Salt and pepper to liking

Directions:

1. Bring the oven to 375 heat setting. Cut the squash, lengthwise, into 4 steaks. Carefully core one side of each squash with a paring knife in a crosshatch pattern.
2. Using a brush, coat with olive oil each side of the steak then season generously with salt and pepper.
3. In an oven-safe, non-stick skillet, bring 2 tablespoons of olive oil to a warm temperature.
4. Place the steaks on the skillet with the cored side down and cook at medium temperature until browned, approximately 5 minutes.

5. Flip and repeat on the other side for about 3 minutes. Place the skillet into the oven to roast the squash for 7 minutes.
6. Take out from the oven, placing on a plate and covering with aluminum foil to keep warm.
7. Using the previously used skillet, add thyme, garlic, and shallot, cooking at medium heat. Stir frequently for about 2 minutes.
8. Add brandy and cook for an additional minute. Next, add paprika and whisk the mixture together for 3 minutes.
9. Add in the yogurt seasoning with salt and pepper. Plate the steaks and spoon the sauce over the top. Garnish with parsley and enjoy!

Nutrition: Calories: 300 Carbohydrates: 46 g Proteins: 5.3 g Fats: 10.6 g

24. **Cauliflower Steak Kicking Corn**

Preparation time: 15 minutes

Cooking time: 35 minutes

Servings: 6

Ingredients:

- 2 tsp capers, drained
- 4 scallions, chopped
- 1 red chili, minced
- ¼ cup vegetable oil
- 2 ears of corn, shucked
- 2 big cauliflower heads
- Salt and pepper to taste

Directions:

1. Heat the oven to 375 degrees. Boil a pot of water, about 4 cups, using the maximum heat setting available. Add corn in the saucepan, cooking approximately 3 minutes or until tender.
2. Drain and allow the corn to cool, then slice the kernels away from the cob. Warm 2 tablespoons of vegetable oil in a skillet.
3. Combine the chili pepper with the oil, cooking for approximately 30 seconds. Next, combine the scallions, sautéing with the chili pepper until soft.

4. Mix in the corn and capers in the skillet and cook for approximately 1 minute to blend the flavors. Then remove from heat.
5. Warm 1 tablespoon of vegetable oil in a skillet. Once warm, begin to place cauliflower steaks to the pan, 2 to 3 at a time.
6. Season to your liking with salt and cook over medium heat for 3 minutes or until lightly browned. Once cooked, slide onto the cookie sheet and repeat the step with the remaining cauliflower.
7. Take the corn mixture and press into the spaces between the florets of the cauliflower. Bake for 25 minutes. Serve warm and enjoy!

Nutrition: Calories: 153 Carbohydrates: 15 g Proteins: 4 g Fats: 10 g

25. Pistachio Watermelon Steak

Preparation time: 15 minutes

Cooking time: 15 minutes

Servings: 4

Ingredients:

- Microgreens
- Pistachios chopped
- Malden sea salt
- 1 tbsp. olive oil, extra virgin
- 1 watermelon
- Salt to taste

Directions:

1. Begin by cutting the ends of the watermelon. Carefully peel the skin from the watermelon along the white outer edge. Slice the watermelon into 4 slices, approximately 2 inches thick.
2. Trim the slices, so they are rectangular in shape approximately 2 x4 inches. Heat a skillet to medium heat add 1 tablespoon of olive oil.
3. Add watermelon steaks and cook until the edges begin to caramelize. Plate and top with pistachios and microgreens. Sprinkle with Malden salt. Serve warm and enjoy!

Nutrition: Calories: 67 Carbohydrates: 3.8 g Proteins: 1.6 g Fats: 5.9 g

26. Tofu Seitan

Preparation time: 15 minutes

Cooking time: 12 minutes

Servings: 6

Ingredients:

- ½ tsp salt
- 1 tsp garlic, powdered
- 2 tsp vegetable broth
- 1 tbsp. onion, powdered

2 tbsp. of the following

- nutritional yeast
- water
- 1 ¼ cup tofu
- 1 ½ cup vital wheat gluten

Directions:

1. Stir together the ingredients above in a bowl until a dough form. Lightly dust the countertop and your hands with wheat gluten.
2. Using the counter service, form a ball out of the dough. Be careful not to knead it because it might make the seitan tough. Once the ball is formed, cut it into 6 equal pieces.
3. Using your fingers press each ball into an oval shape, about 4x6 inches. With a steamer basket placed inside a

big pot, add water into the bottom of the pot and bring it to a rolling boil.

4. Place the seitan into the steamer basket; if they overlap, brush them with oil to prevent them from sticking. Cover and steam for approximately 12 minutes then flip so that both sides steam evenly.

5. Once steamed on both sides, remove and allow cooling for a minimum of 1 hour.

6. The tenders are fully cooked at this point, so you can re-heat them or toss them on the grill with your favorite sauce, or you can eat them cold over leafy greens. Enjoy!

Nutrition: Calories: 159 Carbohydrates: 8 g Proteins: 26 g
Fats: 2 g

27. Stuffed Zucchini

Preparation time: 15 minutes

Cooking time: 25 minutes

Servings: 4

Ingredients:

- 1 ½ cup black beans, drained
- ¼ tsp chili powder

½ of the following:

- sea salt
- cumin, ground
- 1 tsp of the following:
- clove garlic, minced
- red bell pepper, diced
- red onion, diced
- 1 tbsp. olive oil, extra virgin
- 4 medium zucchinis

For the Sauce:

¼ tsp of the following:

- chili powder
- turmeric
- sea salt
- 1 tbsp. Nutritional yeast
- ½ tsp apple cider vinegar

¼ cup of the following:

- water
- raw tahini
- 4 tsp Lemon juice

Directions:

1. Set the oven to 350 heat setting. Slice the knobs off the top and bottom of the zucchini, and then slice in half lengthwise.
2. Scoop the center of the seeds from each zucchini with a spoon, creating a bowl to hold the filling. On a big cookie sheet, place the zucchini bowls and bake for approximately 20 minutes.
3. Using a big skillet, combine onion and pepper and sauté for five minutes at medium-high temperature until softened. Add garlic and sauté for an additional minute.
4. Turn the skillet down to medium heat and sprinkle in the chili powder, cumin, salt, and black beans and warm. Remove from the stove and cover to maintain warmth.
5. Prepare the sauce. Using a little bowl, whisk the sauce ingredients until smooth and creamy. Remove the zucchini from the oven when finished cooking.
6. Fill each zucchini bowl generously with the bean mixture. Drizzle the sauce over. Serve warm and enjoy!

Nutrition: Calories: 159 Carbohydrates: 8 g Proteins: 26 g Fats: 2 g

28. Roasted Butternut Squash with Chimichurri

Preparation time: 15 minutes

Cooking time: 15 minutes

Servings: 2

Ingredients:

- 1 cup onion, thinly sliced
- 2 cloves garlic
- 1 tbsp. coconut oil
- 1 acorn squash
- 2 tbsp. olive oil (best if extra virgin)
- ¼ cup goji berries
- 1 cup water
- 2 cups mushrooms, sliced
- ½ cup quinoa

Chimichurri Sauce:

- ½ tsp salt
- 2 tbsp. lime
- ½ cup olive oil, extra virgin
- ¼ tsp cayenne pepper
- 1 shallot
- 3 cloves garlic
- 1 tbsp. sherry vinegar
- 1 cup parsley

Directions:

1. Bring the broiler to the maximum heat setting. Stir up the chimichurri sauce by combining the parsley, vinegar, garlic shallot, cayenne pepper, olive oil, lime juice, and ½ cup of olive oil.
2. Blend well; if you want the sauce a little thinner, then add additional extra virgin oil. Prepare an aluminum-foiled cookie sheet.
3. Divide the squash in half by carefully cutting widthwise, and remove seeds and pulp from the center. Cut each half of the squash into moon shape slices; you should get about 4-6 slices.
4. Place the slices on the aluminum foil sheet and spritz olive oil across the top. Once one side is charred to your liking, flip the squash and char the other side.
5. While broiling, bring a medium-sized saucepan of water to a rolling boil then simmer the quinoa, cooking for 10 minutes or until tender.
6. Heat a skillet to medium heat, and sauté the onions. Once the onions are caramelizing, add in the mushroom and garlic, cooking on low heat for approximately 5 minutes.
7. Plate the squash, topping it with quinoa and mushroom. Sprinkle goji berries across the plate and drizzle chimichurri sauce. Serve warm and enjoy!

Nutrition: Calories: 615 Carbohydrates: 71.6 g Proteins: 12.5 g Fats: 35.7 g

29. Eggplant Pizza

Preparation time: 15 minutes

Cooking time: 30 minutes

Servings: 8

Ingredients:

- 2 tbsp. olive oil

¼ tsp of the following:

- pepper
- salt
- ½ tsp oregano, dried
- 1 cup panko
- ½ tbsp. almond flour
- 1 tbsp. flaxseed, ground
- 1/3 cup water
- ½ eggplant, medium size
- 2 cups marinara sauce
- 1 lb. vegan pizza dough

For the cheese:

- ¼ lb. tofu, extra firm drained
- 2 tbsp. almond milk, unsweetened
- ½ cup cashews, soaked for 6 hours, drained
- 3 tbsp. lemon juice, freshly squeezed

Directions:

1. Set the oven to 400 heat setting; prepare a cookie sheet with ½ tablespoon of olive oil by brushing to coat. Whisk together flaxseed, flour, and water in a little bowl.

2. In a different bowl, combine salt, pepper, oregano, and panko. Prepare the eggplant by slicing into ¼ inch triangles.

3. Dip each eggplant triangle into the flaxseed mixture then coat with panko mixture and place on the cookie sheet.

4. Slide gently into the oven and baking for 15 minutes. Flip and then bake for an additional 15 minutes or until lightly browned.

5. Take out of the oven and set to the side. Get a pizza stone or pizza pan ready for the dough.

6. Lightly flour the workspace, and with a rolling pin, work the dough to a 14-inch circle then transfer to the pizza stone or pizza pan.

7. Brush the dough's top with olive oil and slide into the warm oven, cooking until lightly browned or for about twenty minutes.

8. While the crust is baking, prepare the cheese by placing cashews in the high-speed blender, blending until it reaches a crumbly consistency.

9. Then add to the blender the lemon juice, almond milk, and tofu; blend until it's a chunky cheese-like consistency. Set to the side.

10. Once the crust is cooked, assemble the pizza by saucing crust with marinara, adding eggplant slices, and placing the cheese on top. Serve warm and enjoy!

Nutrition: Calories: 234 Carbohydrates: 27 g Proteins: 5.4 g Fats: 12 g

30. Green Avocado Carbonara

Preparation time: 15 minutes

Cooking time: 0 minutes

Servings: 1

Ingredients:

- Spinach angel hair
- Parsley, fresh
- 2 tsp olive oil, extra virgin
- 2 cloves garlic, diced
- ½ lemon, zest, and juice
- 1 avocado, pitted
- Salt and pepper to taste

Directions:

1. Combine using a food processor the parsley, olive oil, garlic, lemon, and avocado and blend until smooth. Prepare the noodles according to package.
2. Place noodles in a bowl, and add the sauce on top of noodles. Add pepper and salt to your liking. Serve warm and enjoy!

Nutrition: Calories: 526 Carbohydrates: 24.6 g Proteins: 5.8 g Fats: 48.7 g

SNACKS

31. Roasted Beetroot Noodles

Preparation Time: 15 minutes

Cooking Time: 20 minutes

Servings: 4

Ingredients:

- 1 tsp orange zest
- 2 tbsp. of the following:
- Parsley, chopped
- Balsamic vinegar
- Olive oil
- 2 big beets, peeled and spiraled

Directions:

1. Set the oven to 425 high-heat settings. In a big bowl, combine the beet noodles, olive oil, and vinegar. Toss until well combined. Season with pepper and salt.
2. Line a big cookie sheet using parchment paper, and spread the noodles out into a single layer. Roast the noodles for 20 minutes.
3. Place into bowls and zest with orange and sprinkle parsley. Gently toss and serve.

Nutrition: Calories: 44 Protein: 2.71 g Fat: 1.71 g
Carbohydrates: 5.02 g

32. **Turnip Fries**

Preparation Time: 25 minutes

Cooking Time: 20 minutes

Servings: 8

Ingredients:

- 1 tsp. onion powder
- 1 tsp. paprika
- 1 tsp. garlic salt
- 1 tbsp. vegetable oil
- 3 pounds turnips

Directions:

1. Set the oven to 425 heat setting. Prepare a lightly greased aluminum foil-lined cookie sheet
2. Using a hand peeler, peel the turnips. With a Mandolin, cut the turnips into French fry sticks. Then place in a big bowl.
3. Toss the turnips with oil to coat then season with onion powder, paprika, and garlic and coat again. Spread evenly across the cookie sheet.
4. Bake for at least 20 minutes or until the outside is crisp. Serve with your favorite sauce or enjoy alone.

Nutrition: Calories: 87 Protein: 5.98 g Fat: 3.15 g
Carbohydrates: 8.76 g

33. Lime and Chili Carrots Noodles

Preparation Time: 10 minutes

Cooking Time: 0 minutes

Servings: 4

Ingredients:

½ tsp of the following:

- Black pepper
- Salt
- 2 tbsp. coconut oil
- ¼ cup coriander, finely chopped
- 2 Jalapeno chilis
- 1 tbsp. lime juice
- 2 carrots, peeled and spiralized

Directions:

1. In a little bowl, combine jalapeno, lime juice, and coconut oil to form a sauce. In a big bowl, place the carrot noodles and pour dressing over the top.
2. Toss to ensure the dressing fully coats the noodles. Season with pepper and salt. Serve and enjoy.

Nutrition: Calories: 93 Protein: 1.92 g Fat: 8.4 g
Carbohydrates: 3.28 g

34. Pesto Zucchini Noodles

Preparation Time: 15 minutes

Cooking Time: 0 minutes

Servings: 4

Ingredients:

- 4 little zucchini ends trimmed
- Cherry tomatoes
- 2 tsp fresh lemon juice
- 1/3 cup olive oil (best if extra-virgin)
- 2 cups packed basil leaves
- 2 cups garlic
- Salt and pepper to taste

Directions:

1. Spiral zucchini into noodles and set to the side. In a food processor, put the basil and garlic and chop. Slowly add olive oil while chopping. Then pulse blend it until thoroughly mixed.
2. In a big bowl, place the noodles and pour pesto sauce over the top. Toss to combine. Garnish with tomatoes and serve and enjoy.

Nutrition: Calories: 173 Protein: 8.63 g Fat: 3.7 g
Carbohydrates: 30.52 g

35. Cabbage Slaw

Preparation Time: 2 hours 5 minutes

Cooking Time: 0 minutes

Servings: 6

Ingredients:

- 1/8 tsp celery seed
- ¼ tsp salt
- 2 tbsp. of the following:
- Apple cider vinegar
- Sweetener of your choice
- ½ cup vegan mayo
- 4 cups coleslaw mix with red cabbage and carrots

Directions:

1. In a big mixing bowl, put and whisk together the celery seed, salt, apple cider vinegar, sweetener, and vegan mayo.
2. Add the coleslaw and stir until appropriately combined. Refrigerate while covered for a minimum of 2 hours or overnight if you're not in a hurry. Garnish with tomatoes and serve and enjoy.

Nutrition: Calories: 136 Protein: 4.63 g Fat: 1.88 g
Carbohydrates: 29.77 g

36. Avocado Sandwich

Preparation Time: 5 Minutes

Cooking Time: 5 Minutes

Servings: 2

Ingredients:

- 8 whole-wheat bread slices
- ½ oz. vegan butter
- 2 oz. little gem lettuce, cleaned and patted dry
- 1 oz. tofu cheese, sliced
- 1 avocado, pitted, peeled, and sliced
- 1 small cucumber, sliced into 4 rings
- Freshly chopped parsley to garnish

Directions:

1. Arrange the 4 bread slices on a flat surface and smear the vegan butter on one end each. Place a lettuce leaf on each and arrange some tofu cheese on top. Top with the avocado and cucumber slices.
2. Garnish the sandwiches with a little parsley, cover with the remaining bread slices, and serve immediately.

Nutrition: Calories: 380 Fat: 21g Carbs: 44g Protein: 9.0g

37. Tacos

Preparation Time: 10 Minutes

Cooking Time: 30 Minutes

Servings: 4

Ingredients:

- 6 Taco Shells

For the slaw:

- 1 cup Red Cabbage, shredded
- 3 Scallions, chopped
- 1 cup Green Cabbage, shredded
- 1 cup Carrots, sliced

For the dressing:

- 1 tbsp. Sriracha
- ¼ cup Apple Cider Vinegar
- ¼ tsp. Salt
- 2 tbsp. Sesame Oil
- 1 tbsp. Dijon Mustard
- 1 tbsp. Lime Juice
- ½ tbsp. Tamari
- 1 tbsp. Maple Syrup
- ¼ tsp. Salt

Directions:

1. For the dressing, put and whisk all the ingredients in a small bowl until mixed well. Next, combine the slaw ingredients in another bowl and toss well.
2. Finally, take a taco shell and place the slaw in it. Serve and enjoy.

Nutrition: Calories: 216 Protein: 10g Carbohydrates: 15g Fat: 13g

38. Cheese Cucumber Bites

Preparation Time: 10 minutes

Cooking Time: 0 minutes

Servings: 8

Ingredients:

- 4 large cucumbers
- 1 cup raw sunflower seeds
- 1/2 tsp salt
- 2 tbsp. raw red onion, chopped
- 1 handful fresh chives, chopped
- 1 clove fresh garlic, chopped
- 2 tbsp. nutritional yeast
- 2 tbsp. fresh lemon juice
- 1/2 cup water

Directions:

1. Start by blending sunflower seeds with salt in a food processor for 20 seconds. Toss in remaining ingredients except for the cucumber and chives and process until smooth.
2. Slice the cucumber into 1.5-inch thick rounds. Top each slice with sunflower mixture. Garnish with sumac and chives. Serve.

Nutrition: Calories 211 Fat 25.5 g Carbs 32.4 g Protein 1.4 g

39. Mango Sticky Rice

Preparation Time: 15 Minutes

Cooking Time: 20 minutes

Servings: 3

Ingredients:

- ½ cup sugar
- 1 mango, sliced
- 14 ounces coconut milk, canned
- ½ cup basmati rice

Directions:

1. Cook your rice per package instructions, and add half of your sugar. When cooking your rice, substitute half of your water for half of your coconut milk.
2. Boil your remaining coconut milk in a saucepan with your remaining sugar. Boil on high heat until it's thick, and then add in your mango slices.

Nutrition: Calories: 571 Protein: 6 g Fat: 29.6 g Carbs: 77.6 g

40. Green Chips

Preparation time: 15 minutes

Cooking time: 10-20 minutes

Servings: 2

Ingredients:

- 2 or 3 large green leaves or 5 or 6 small leaves of kale, cabbage, collards, orchard, washed, dried, stemmed, and torn into small pieces
- 1 tablespoon olive oil
- 1 tablespoon nutritional yeast (optional)
- 1 teaspoon onion powder (optional)
- Pinch salt

Directions:

1. Preheat the oven to 300°F. Put the greens on a rimmed baking sheet, and sprinkle with the olive oil, nutritional yeast (if using), onion powder (if using), and salt.
2. Massage the spices into the leaves. Spread the leaves out in a single layer so they dry evenly. Bake for 10 to 20 minutes, until the greens are crispy and dry.
3. Remove the greens from the oven, and let them sit for a few minutes to cool before serving. Store in an airtight container, though it's best to bake and enjoy them the same day.

Nutrition: Calories: 93 Protein: 2g Fat: 7g Carbohydrates: 7g

DESSERT RECIPES

41. Pumpkin Pie Squares

Preparation time: 15 minutes

Cooking time: 30 minutes

Servings: 16 squares

Ingredients:

- 1 cup unsweetened almond milk
- 1 teaspoon vanilla extract
- 7 ounces dates, pitted and chopped
- 1¼ cups old-fashioned rolled oats
- 2 teaspoons pumpkin pie spice
- 1 (15-ounce) can pure pumpkin

Directions:

1. Warm your oven to 375ºF (190ºC). Put the parchment paper in a baking pan. Stir together the milk and vanilla in a bowl. Soak the dates in it for 15 minutes, or until the dates become softened.
2. Add the rolled oats to a food processor and pulse the oats into flour. Remove the oat flour from the food processor bowl and whisk together with the pumpkin pie spice in a different bowl.
3. Place the milk mixture into the food processor and process until smooth. Add the flour mixture and

pumpkin to the food processor and pulse until the mixture has broken down into a chunky paste consistency.

4. Transfer the batter to the prepared pan and smooth the top with a silicone spatula. Bake within 30 minutes, or until a toothpick inserted in the center of the pie comes out clean. Let cool completely before cutting into squares. Serve cold.

Nutrition: Calories: 68 Fat: 0.9g Carbs: 16.8g Protein: 2.3g

42. Apple Crisp

Preparation time: 15 minutes

Cooking time: 40 minutes

Servings: 6

Ingredients:

- ½ cup vegan butter
- 6 large apples, diced large
- 1 cup dried cranberries
- 2 tablespoons granulated sugar
- 2 teaspoons ground cinnamon, divided
- ¼ teaspoon ground nutmeg
- ¼ teaspoon ground ginger
- 2 teaspoons lemon juice
- 1 cup all-purpose flour
- 1 cup rolled oats
- 1 cup brown sugar
- ¼ teaspoon salt

Directions:

1. Preheat the oven to 350°F. Oiled an 8-inch square baking dish with butter or cooking spray.
2. Make the filling. In a large bowl, combine the apples, cranberries, granulated sugar, 1 teaspoon of cinnamon, the nutmeg, ginger, and lemon juice. Toss to coat. Transfer the apple mixture to the prepared baking dish.

3. Make the topping. In the same large bowl, now empty, combine the all-purpose flour, oats, brown sugar, and salt. Stir to combine.
4. Add the butter and, using a pastry cutter (or two knives moving in a crisscross pattern), cut the butter into the flour and oat mixture until the butter is the size of small peas.
5. Spread the topping over the apples evenly, patting down slightly. Bake for 40 minutes or until golden and bubbly.

Nutrition: Calories: 488 Fat: 9 g Carbs: 101 g Protein: 5 g

43. Secret Ingredient Chocolate Brownies

Preparation time: 15 minutes

Cooking time: 35 minutes

Servings: 6-8

Ingredients:

- ¾ cup flour
- ¼ teaspoon baking soda
- ¼ teaspoon salt
- 1/3 cup vegan butter
- ¾ cup sugar
- 2 tablespoon water
- 1¼ cups semi-sweet or dark dairy-free chocolate chips
- 6 tablespoons aquafaba, divided
- 1 teaspoon vanilla extract

Directions:

1. Preheat the oven to 325°F. Line a 9-inch square baking pan with parchment or grease well. In a large bowl, combine the flour, baking soda, and salt. Set aside.
2. In a medium saucepan over medium-high heat, combine the butter, sugar, and water. Bring to a boil, stirring occasionally. Remove then stir in the chocolate chips.

3. Whisk in 3 tablespoons of aquafaba until thoroughly combined. Add the vanilla extract and the remaining 3 tablespoons of aquafaba, and whisk until mixed.
4. Add the chocolate mixture into the flour mixture and stir until combined. Pour in an even layer into the prepared pan.
5. Bake for 35 minutes, until the top is set but the brownie jiggles slightly when shaken. Allow to cool completely, 45 minutes to 1 hour, before removing and serving.

Nutrition: Calories: 369 Fat: 19 g Carbs: 48 g Protein: 4 g

44. Chocolate Chip Pecan Cookies

Preparation time: 15 minutes

Cooking time: 16 minutes

Servings: 30 cookies

Ingredients:

- ¾ cup pecan halves, toasted
- 1 cup vegan butter
- ½ teaspoon salt
- ½ cup powdered sugar
- 2 teaspoons vanilla extract
- 2 cups all-purpose flour
- 1 cup mini dairy-free chocolate chips, such as Enjoy Life brand

Directions:

1. Preheat the oven to 350°F. Prepare a large rimmed baking sheet lined using parchment paper.
2. In a small skillet over medium heat, toast the pecans until warm and fragrant, about 2 minutes. Remove from the pan. Once these are cool, chop them into small pieces.
3. Combine the butter, salt, and powdered sugar, and cream using an electric hand mixer or a stand mixer fitted with a paddle attachment on high speed for 3 to 4 minutes, until light and fluffy. Add the vanilla extract and beat for 1 minute.

4. Turn the mixer on low and slowly add the flour, ½ cup at a time, until a dough form. Put the chocolate chips plus pecans, and mix until just incorporated.
5. Using your hands, a large spoon, or a 1-inch ice cream scoop, drop 1-inch balls of dough on the baking sheet, spaced 1 inch apart. Gently press down on the cookies to flatten them slightly.
6. Bake for 12 to 14 minutes until just golden around the edges. Cool on the baking sheet within 5 minutes before transferring them to a wire rack to cool. Serve or store in an airtight container.

Nutrition: Calories: 152 Fat: 11 g Carbs: 13 g Protein: 2 g

45. Peanut Butter Chip Cookies

Preparation time: 15 minutes

Cooking time: 15 minutes

Servings: 12-15

Ingredients:

- 1 tablespoon ground flaxseed
- 3 tablespoons hot water
- 1 cup rolled oats
- 1 teaspoon baking soda
- 1 teaspoon ground cinnamon
- ¼ teaspoon salt
- 1 ripe banana, mashed
- ¼ cup maple syrup
- ½ cup all-natural smooth peanut butter
- 1 tablespoon vanilla extract
- ½ cup dairy-free chocolate chips

Directions:

1. Preheat the oven to 350°F. Prepare a large rimmed baking sheet lined using parchment paper.
2. Make a flaxseed egg by combining the ground flaxseed and hot water in a small bowl. Stir and let it sit for 5 minutes until thickened.
3. In a medium bowl, combine the oats, baking soda, cinnamon, and salt. Set aside.

4. Mash the banana then put the maple syrup, peanut butter, flaxseed egg, and vanilla extract in a large bowl. Stir to combine.
5. Add the dry batter into the wet batter and stir until just incorporated (do not overmix). Gently fold in the chocolate chips.
6. Using a large spoon or 2-inch ice cream scoop, drop the cookie dough balls onto the baking sheet. Flatten them slightly.
7. Bake within 12 to 15 minutes or until the bottoms and edges are slightly browned. Serve or store in an airtight container.

Nutrition: Calories: 192 Fat: 12 g Carbs: 17 g Protein: 6 g

46. No-Bake Chocolate Coconut Energy Balls

Preparation time: 15 minutes

Cooking time: 0 minutes

Servings: 9

Ingredients:

- ¼ cup dry roasted or raw pumpkin seeds
- ¼ cup dry roasted or raw sunflower seeds
- ½ cup unsweetened shredded coconut
- 2 tablespoons chia seeds
- ¼ teaspoon salt
- 1½ tablespoons Dutch process cocoa powder
- ¼ cup rolled oats
- 2 tablespoons coconut oil, melted
- 6 pitted dates
- 2 tablespoons all-natural almond butter

Directions:

1. Combine the pumpkin seeds, sunflower seeds, coconut, chia seeds, salt, cocoa powder, and oats in a food processor or blender. Pulse until the mix is coarsely crumbled.
2. Add the coconut oil, dates, and almond butter. Pulse until the batter is combined and sticks when squeezed between your fingers.

3. Scoop out 2 tablespoons of mix at a time and roll them into 1½-inch balls with your hands. Place them spaced apart on a freezer-safe plate and freeze for 15 minutes.
4. Remove from the freezer and keep refrigerated in an airtight container for up to 4 days.

Nutrition: Calories: 230 Fat: 12 g Carbs: 27 g Protein: 5 g

47. Blueberry Hand Pies

Preparation time: 15 minutes

Cooking time: 20 minutes

Servings: 6-8

Ingredients:

- 3 cups all-purpose flour, + extra for dusting work surface
- ½ teaspoon salt
- ¼ cup, plus 2 tablespoons granulated sugar, divided
- 1 cup vegan butter
- ½ cup cold water
- 1 cup fresh blueberries
- 2 teaspoons lemon zest
- 2 teaspoons lemon juice
- ¼ teaspoon ground cinnamon
- 1 teaspoon cornstarch
- ¼ cup unsweetened soy milk
- Coarse sugar, for sprinkling

Directions:

1. Warm your oven to 375°F. Prepare a large baking sheet lined using parchment paper. Set aside.
2. In a large bowl, combine the flour, salt, 2 tablespoons of granulated sugar, and vegan butter. Using a pastry cutter or two knives moving in a crisscross pattern, cut

the butter into the other ingredients until the butter is the size of small peas.

3. Put the cold water then knead to form a dough. Tear the dough in half and wrap the halves separately in plastic wrap. Refrigerate for 15 minutes.

4. Make the blueberry filling. In a medium bowl, combine the blueberries, lemon zest, lemon juice, cinnamon, cornstarch, and the remaining ¼ cup of sugar.

5. Remove one half of the dough. On a floured surface, roll out the dough to ¼- to ½-inch thickness. Turn a 5-inch bowl upside down, and, using it as a guide, cut the dough into circles to make mini pie crusts.

6. Reroll scrap dough to cut out more circles. Repeat with the second half of the dough. You should end up with 10 to 12 circles. Place the circles on the prepared sheet pan.

7. Spoon 1½ tablespoons of blueberry filling onto each circle, leaving a ¼-inch border. Fold the circles in half to cover the filling, forming a half-moon shape. Press the edges of your dough to seal the pies using a fork.

8. When all the pies are assembled, use a paring knife to score the pies by cutting three lines through the top crusts.

9. Brush each pie with soy milk and sprinkle with coarse sugar. Bake for 20 minutes or until the filling is bubbly and the tops are golden. Let cool before serving.

Nutrition: Calories: 416 Fat: 23 g Carbs: 46 g Protein: 6 g

48. Date Squares

Preparation time: 15 minutes

Cooking time: 25 minutes

Servings: 12

Ingredients:

- Cooking spray, for greasing
- 1½ cups rolled oats
- 1½ cups all-purpose flour
- ¾ cup, + 1/3 cup brown sugar, divided
- ½ teaspoon ground cinnamon
- ¼ teaspoon ground nutmeg
- 1 teaspoon baking soda
- ¼ teaspoon salt
- ¾ cup vegan butter
- 18 pitted dates
- 1 teaspoon lemon zest
- 1 teaspoon lemon juice
- 1 cup water

Directions:

1. Preheat the oven to 350°F. Oiled or spray a 9-inch square baking dish. Set aside.
2. Make the base and topping mixture. In a large bowl, combine the rolled oats, flour, ¾ cup of brown sugar, cinnamon, nutmeg, baking soda, and salt.

3. Add the butter and, using a pastry cutter or two knives working in a crisscross motion, cut the butter into the mixture to form a crumbly dough. Press half of your dough into the prepared baking dish and set the remaining half aside.
4. For the date filling, place a small saucepan over medium heat. Add the dates, the remaining 1/3 cup of sugar, the lemon zest, lemon juice, and water. Boil and cook within 7 to 10 minutes, until thickened.
5. When cooked, pour the date mixture over the dough base in the baking dish and top with the remaining crumb dough.
6. Gently press down and spread evenly to cover all the filling. Bake for 25 minutes until lightly golden on top. Cool before serving. Store in an airtight container.

Nutrition: Calories: 443 Fat: 12 g Carbs: 81 g Protein: 5 g

49. Crazy Chocolate Cake

Preparation time: 15 minutes

Cooking time: 35 minutes

Servings: 12

Ingredients:

For the cake:

- Cooking spray, for greasing
- 1½ cups all-purpose flour
- 1 cup granulated sugar
- ¼ cup Dutch process cocoa powder
- 1 teaspoon baking soda
- ½ teaspoon salt
- 1 teaspoon white vinegar
- 5 tablespoons vegetable oil
- 1 teaspoon vanilla extract
- 1 cup water

For the frosting:

- 6 cups powdered sugar
- 1 cup cocoa powder
- 2 cups vegan butter, softened
- 1 teaspoon vanilla extract
- 1 pinch salt

Directions:

1. For the cake, warm your oven to 350°F. Grease or spray an 8-inch square baking dish or a 9-inch round cake pan.
2. In a large bowl, combine the flour, sugar, cocoa powder, baking soda, and salt. Add the vinegar, vegetable oil, vanilla extract, and water directly to the dry ingredients. Stir the batter until no lumps remain.
3. Put the batter into the greased dish and bake for 35 minutes or until a toothpick inserted into the center comes out clean.
4. Once the cake is baked, cool it in the pan for 10 minutes. Transfer it to a plate and refrigerate for about 30 minutes, then frost.
5. For the frosting, mix the powdered sugar plus cocoa powder in a large bowl. Beat the vegan butter on medium-high speed until pale and creamy using an electric hand mixer or a stand mixer with the paddle attachment.
6. Reduce the mixer speed to medium and add the powdered sugar and cocoa mix, ½ cup at a time, mixing well between each addition (about 5 minutes total). Add the vanilla extract and salt and mix on high speed for 1 minute.

Nutrition: Calories: 831 Fat: 44 g Carbs: 111 g Protein: 5 g

50. Chunky Chocolate Peanut Butter Balls

Preparation time: 15 minutes

Cooking time: 0 minutes

Servings: 6

Ingredients:

- ½ cup crunchy peanut butter
- 1½ cups shredded coconut, divided
- 1 cup rolled oats
- ½ cup ground flaxseed
- ¼ cup chia seeds
- ½ cup dairy-free mini chocolate chips
- 1/3 cup maple syrup
- 1 teaspoon vanilla extract

Directions:

1. Melt the peanut butter in a microwave-safe dish for 15 to 20 seconds. In a large bowl, combine 1 cup of the shredded coconut, the rolled oats, ground flaxseed, chia seeds, and chocolate chips.
2. Pour in the melted peanut butter, maple syrup, and vanilla extract. Stir well to combine. Refrigerate within 15 to 20 minutes, until chilled enough that the mixture sticks together when pressed but not so cold that the peanut butter hardens.

3. Place the remaining ½ cup of shredded coconut into a shallow dish. Spoon out 2 tablespoons of the mixture at a time and roll into 1-inch balls.
4. Roll the balls in the remaining ½ cup of shredded coconut to coat. Refrigerate for up to a week.

Nutrition: Calories: 528 Fat: 35 g Carbs: 47 g Protein: 12 g

CONCLUSION

The plant based diet has been picking up in popularity and for good reasons. Studies have shown that people who eat more plant based food can live longer, keep a very healthy weight, reduce the risk of many chronic diseases and even enjoy a better quality of life. There are many good reasons to begin or continue to incorporate more plant based foods into your diet. Plant based foods offer a number of benefits including: being low in calories, low in fat and cholesterol; high in fiber with soluble fiber having a lower glycemic index than starch or sugar; high in antioxidants which protect against degenerative diseases; and low in saturated fat and sodium levels.

The goals of the Boston Vegetarians are to promote a plant based healthy lifestyle through education, enhancing our members' lives through online social networking, creating innovative educational resources and serving as an advocate for ethical, sustainable food production as related to the natural environment.

Going on a plant-based diet means cutting out meat, which cuts away the risks associated with meat. According to the American Heart Association, removing or reducing meat intake from your diet reduces the risk of stroke, high cholesterol, high blood pressure, cancer, diabetes, and obesity.

The AHA also conducted a study back in 2019, and they discovered that middle-aged adults whose diet consists primarily of plants and low amounts of animal products have a low risk of heart disease.

A plant-based diet is also useful for those who already have diabetes. As mentioned before, it helps manage or even prevent diabetes altogether by improving your insulin sensitivity and reducing insulin resistance.

Bad insulin sensitivity and strong insulin resistance mean that the insulin your body produces does not work as it should, which warrants more insulin administration via shots. When you take those problems away by changing your diet, you can be free from diabetes and not rely on insulin shots.

CPSIA information can be obtained
at www.ICGtesting.com
Printed in the USA
BVHW010853250621
610445BV00002B/102

Rapid Weight Loss Hypnosis for Women

A Complete Guide to Losing Weight Fast with Hypnosis, Meditation, and Healthy Eating Habits

DIANA WILLIAMS

Copyright © 2021 by Diana Williams
All rights reserved.

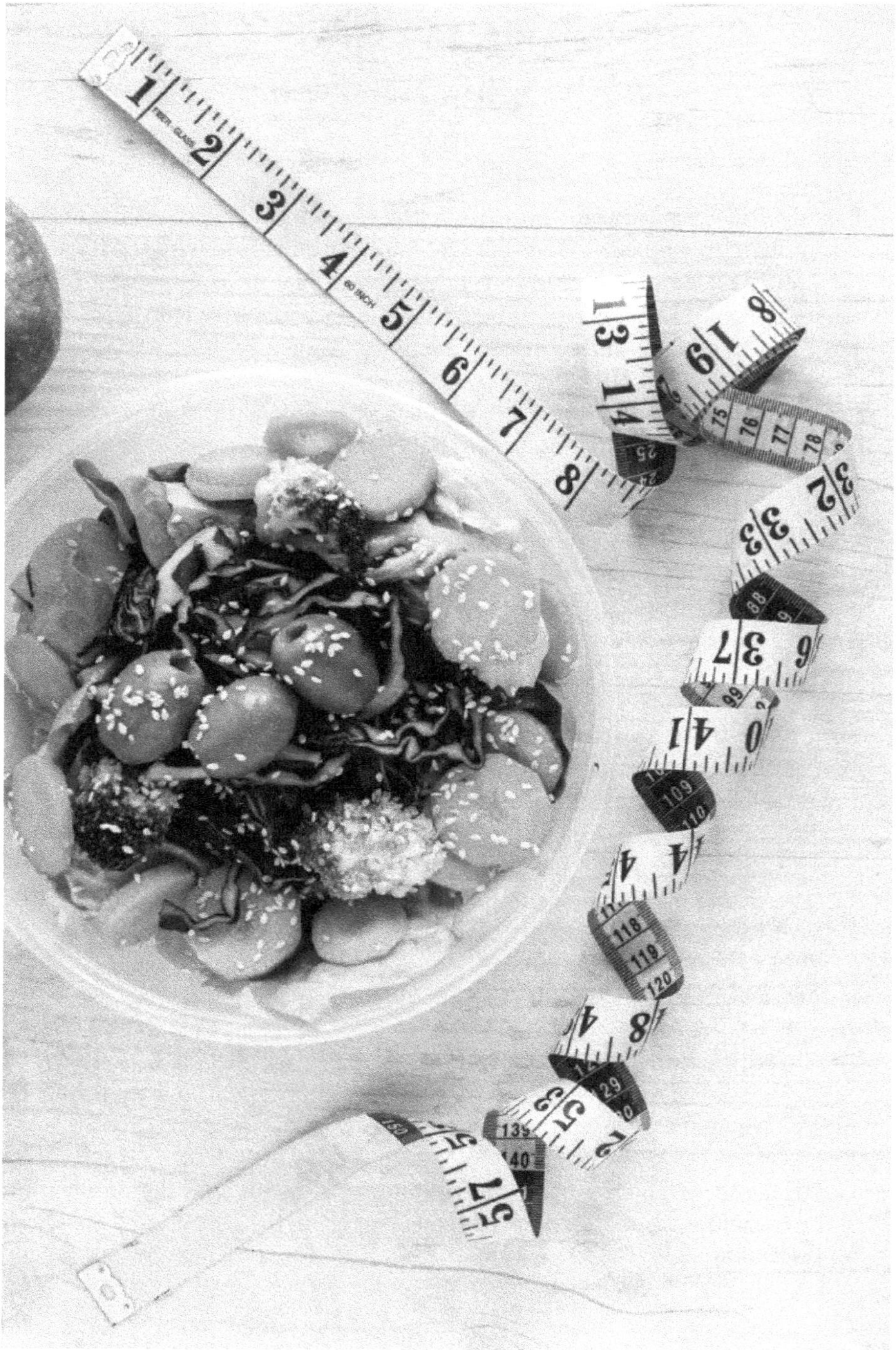

DISCLAIMER

Weight loss results vary from person to person. This book is not intended as a substitute for the medical advice of physicians. The reader should regularly consult a physician in matters relating to his/her health and particularly with respect to any symptoms that may require diagnosis or medical attention. The content on this book is for informational purposes only.

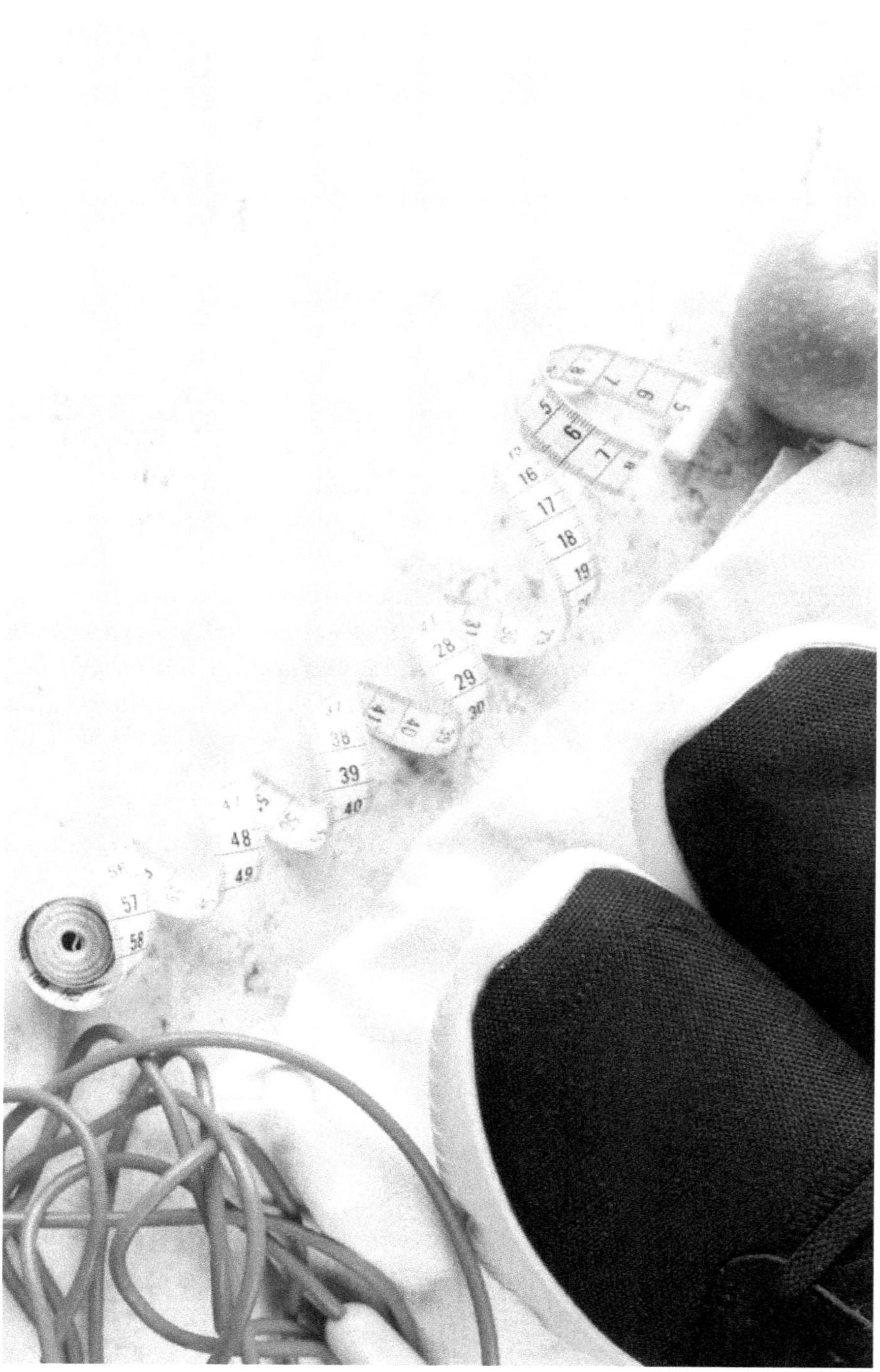

Table of Contents

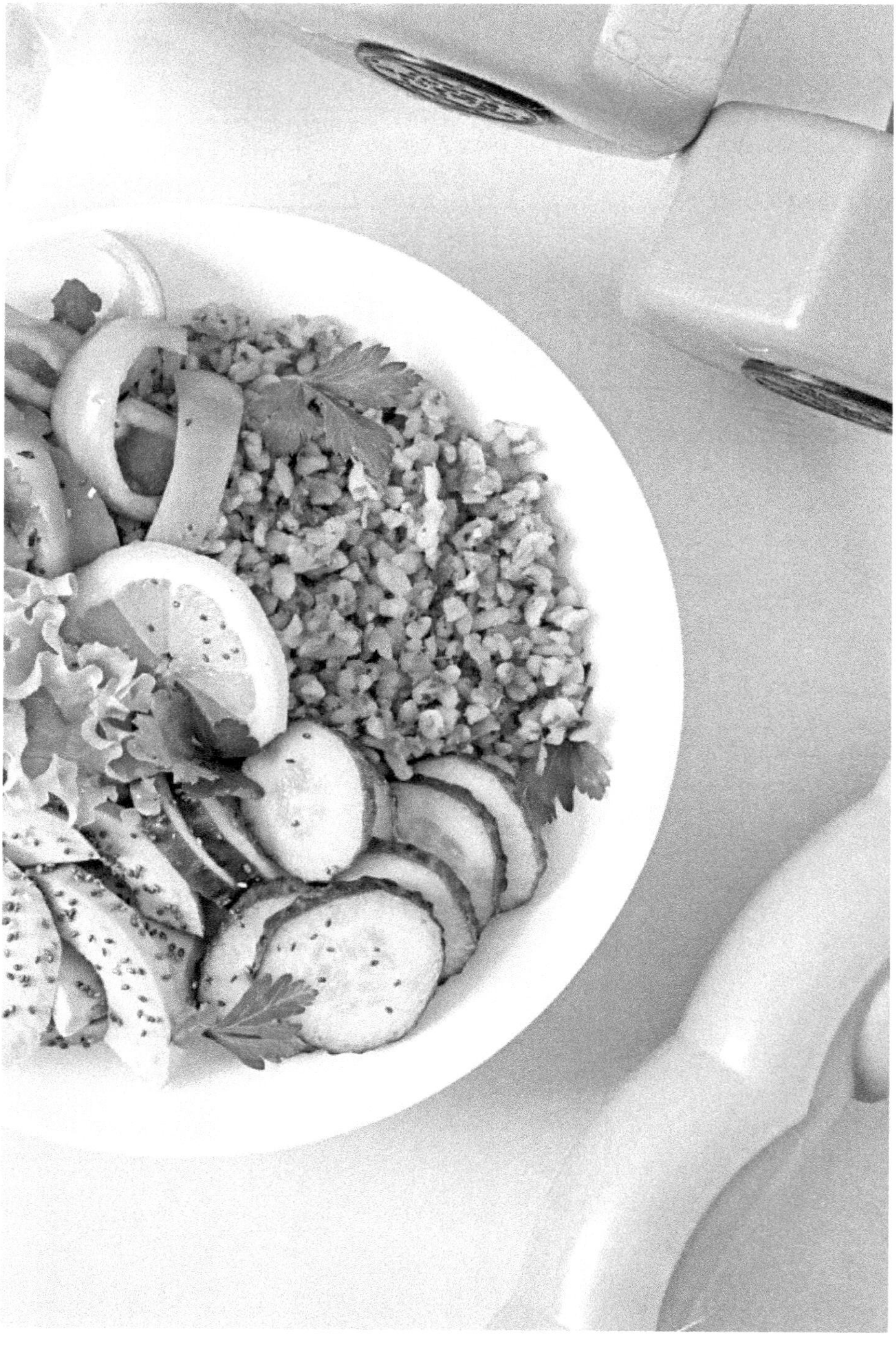

Introduction

Several people have found out that with the aid of hypnotherapy for fast weight loss, they might effectively shed pounds based on their preference.

Using self-hypnosis to lose weight may likely profit you in different ways. To begin with, it will let you develop a completely new self-image. You will possibly develop the self-assurance which you will need to be a person who has the authority to reach your goals; once you have already attained your fast weight loss efforts, your self-confidence will continue to develop.

Hypnosis for weight loss is a precious tool in your diet and exercise arsenal. By using hypnosis daily, you can lose the pounds and gain control of your weight once and for all. Hypnosis has the potential to improve not only your weight but also every area of your life.

By learning about hypnosis, you can see all of the good it will do. It will change your entire outlook.

Although there is much talk about hypnosis for weight loss, it can work if you have other areas that you wish to work on. If you are shy, hypnosis can help you speak in front of large crowds with ease. If you tend to procrastinate, this can give you the motivation you need to get started on a project.

Self-hypnosis can work for almost anything, and you can learn to do this on your own; it just takes time and practice. Some do have concerns that this is a form of mind control.

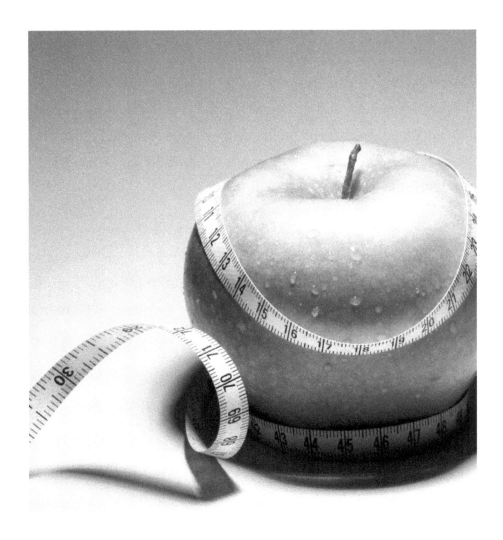

Chapter 1.

Find Your Motivation for Weight Loss and Feel More Energy

If you want to succeed at slimming, motivation will be the most important part you will have to work at. It will give you the determination to get up and exercise even if we don't feel like it.

Motivation is thus an important deciding factor for our success in our weight loss effort. Motivation levels vary from person to person and from day today.

The quality of your inspiration will decide how effective you're in your weight reduction endeavors. The more you advance and reduce, the harder it'll be to lose further because the body is pushed past its natural set points. It's possible to realize remarkable results when a person's motivation is high.

The secret of losing weight is your craving to try it badly enough and find the motivation to ascertain the plan through and realize your goal. Begin by asking this easy but important question, "Who am I losing weight for?" Your answer, which can surely be, "Me" will offer you the needed motivation.

Always bear in mind the benefits of losing weight; that way, you'll not lose sight of your motivation. Write a list of how you would feel when your extra pounds are shed.

You could enlist ideas like: look so smart and sexy in your jeans; feel more confident; feel good about yourself; await occasions to wear that hip clinging, low neck dress; the list could be endless.

Those who have lost weight say that they feel more confident, their health has improved, they get more attention from people,are more energetic and get better and more job opportunities.

If you have no fear of reaching your weight loss goals, your weight loss motivation will work. Forget any negativity and focus on weight loss benefits of having more energy, a stronger heart, breathing better, and setting a good example for others. Focusing on the objective and your destination will give you the needed motivation to stay on the right track with continued motivation.

A prevalent reason for people to lose interest in exercise and dieting is due to unrealistic goals set by them. When we see images of perfect bodies in the media or on television together with the false promises that their messages give, we too feel that we can and must have a body like that after using the merchandise advertised; when this does not happen, we feel we've failed and believe we cannot reach the specified goal then give up.

Don't forget the time it took to realize the weight; that way, you will not expect to break down any faster. As you start losing weight, you will be flooded with compliments - this, in turn, will help keep you motivated. If you want to lose weight and have enough support to help you in this cause, you'll achieve your goal.

Stay Motivated for Weight Loss

Staying motivated is crucial to complete your weight loss program successfully. Often, in the first week of your weight loss program, you are very excited and do whatever you can to lose weight. You go to the gym;you change your eating habits; and you get up early in the morning and go for a walk. The first week goes on great.

In the second week, your old habits win over your new habits. You go to a lunchroom with your companions and can't prevent yourself from eating that fiery burgers and pizzas and so on.You won't even feel like going to the gym. You show idleness in getting up early in the morning as well.

Why does all this happen? We are super excited in the first few weeks, and then in the next few weeks, all our energy and excitement vanishes, and we finally give up.

The answer is simple. It's all because of a Lack of Motivation. We are super motivated in the first week of our weight loss endeavor.

Inspiration prompts vitality and fervor, which thusly encourages us to do all that we can to lose weight. In any case, in the subsequent week, our inspiration begins to back off, and, accordingly, we want to stop, surrendering, and return to our old propensities.

It's all because of Low Motivation that most people often quit on their weight loss program. You can keep yourself motivated during rough spots using Motivational Quotes.

Tips and Advice to Motivate Yourself to Lose Weight

One of the main difficulties, when you want to lose weight, is to find the motivation to do so.

How many of us have embarked on regimes that we did not keep for lack of real motivation or sufficient strength of character to face this challenge?

Losing weight is not trivial, and above all, it is not easy. More often than not, having a lack of motivation has more to do with the structure of our weight loss program than with the mentality that we have.

❖ Motivation to Lose Weight: Ask Yourself the Right Questions

Before embarking on a slimming cure, you will have to ask yourself why you are doing it—a simple question, which many do not ask.

It happens that we start a diet after reflecting a loved one who pointed out our apparent little can, or of our mother. She tells us that we should be a bit careful about what we eat . This may be due to reading papers in which stunning fine women appear, making you want to look like them to seduce.

But if you have to lose weight effectively, it is mainly for yourself. And to keep your motivation to lose weight, you have to be highly interested!

If you realize that you are not doing it for yourself, it will undoubtedly be more difficult to stick to your diet because of someone else.

On the other hand, if you decide to regain control and eliminate your extra pounds for good reasons (aesthetics, health, and more), and all these are important to you, then you are already on a good footing.

❖ Think About the Negative Consequences

When you have low motivation and want to snack or eat something unhealthy, you are too lazy to do your workout.

Rather than thinking about the positive sides of the action: instant satisfaction, eating something sweet, staying quiet at home, etc., think of the negative consequences: we are going to screw up a day of effort, we will take more time to reach our objectives, we will have to make efforts for longer, etc.

❖ Imagine Realizing Your New Habits

No matter what project you want to do, it's all about habits. And in the end, it is they who make all the difference.

The problem with habits is that we have to manage to incorporate them sustainably into our daily lives. To do this, you have to imagine yourself carrying out the actions that make up this habit.

The more details, the more effective it will be.

When you have the idea of a habit that will help you advance your project, imagine yourself carrying it out.

So when the real-time comes to perform this action, you will have no more problems since your brain will already be prepared to perform it, it will already be somewhat used to it.

❖ Compare the Two Possible Futures

To achieve what you want to achieve, you have to make the right choices. Easy to say, but day today, it is not easy not to crack. And that's why we have to project ourselves into the future.

When one is faced with a desire, or on the contrary, it is necessary to compare the two possible futures with laziness. See yourself in a situation where you make the wrong choice and the one where you make the right choice.

Imagine the consequences of your actions, and you will see that you will always make the right decision. This little exercise will help you take action when necessary and not crack when you are subjected to temptation.

❖ Understand That It Is Only Starting That Is Difficult

It is always the beginning, the start, which is the most difficult. Who once said to himself at the gym: "damn, it pisses me off to be here." Who once said to himself after cooking a healthy dish: "it annoys me to eat that." On the contrary, we are happy and proud to have moved and to have accomplished something during our day. In reality, all the difficulty is in starting. Once we have passed that, it's easy; everything is done on its own, without effort.

So keep that in mind, when you are becoming a little lazy: you are already doing the most difficult part. If you pass this test, the rest will flow calmly.

❖ Always Keep Your Goals in Mind

Regardless of what you do, there is consistently at least one reason you do it: goals and goals. And these goals are doubly important. First, they help you define the actions you will need to take to get there. Second, they will help you stay motivated for the time it takes to complete your projects.

And that's why you have to keep them in mind, visualize them well. Because when you have lower motivation, you can remember these goals. And they will help you to hold on, to cope. And then, you will be much more likely to make the right choice.

❖ Organize To Overcome Procrastination

Procrastination is everyone's enemy. It is what blocks us in almost everything we want to achieve in life. Fortunately, for us, there are ways to short-circuit it. The first thing to understand is that it is normal to tend to procrastinate. It comes from the very structure of our brain—so no need to lament.

The second thing to understand is that if procrastination is more and more present, it is because it is linked to concentration.

And as we are constantly called upon by our smartphones, our notifications, our emails, etc.,we find it harder and harder to concentrate.

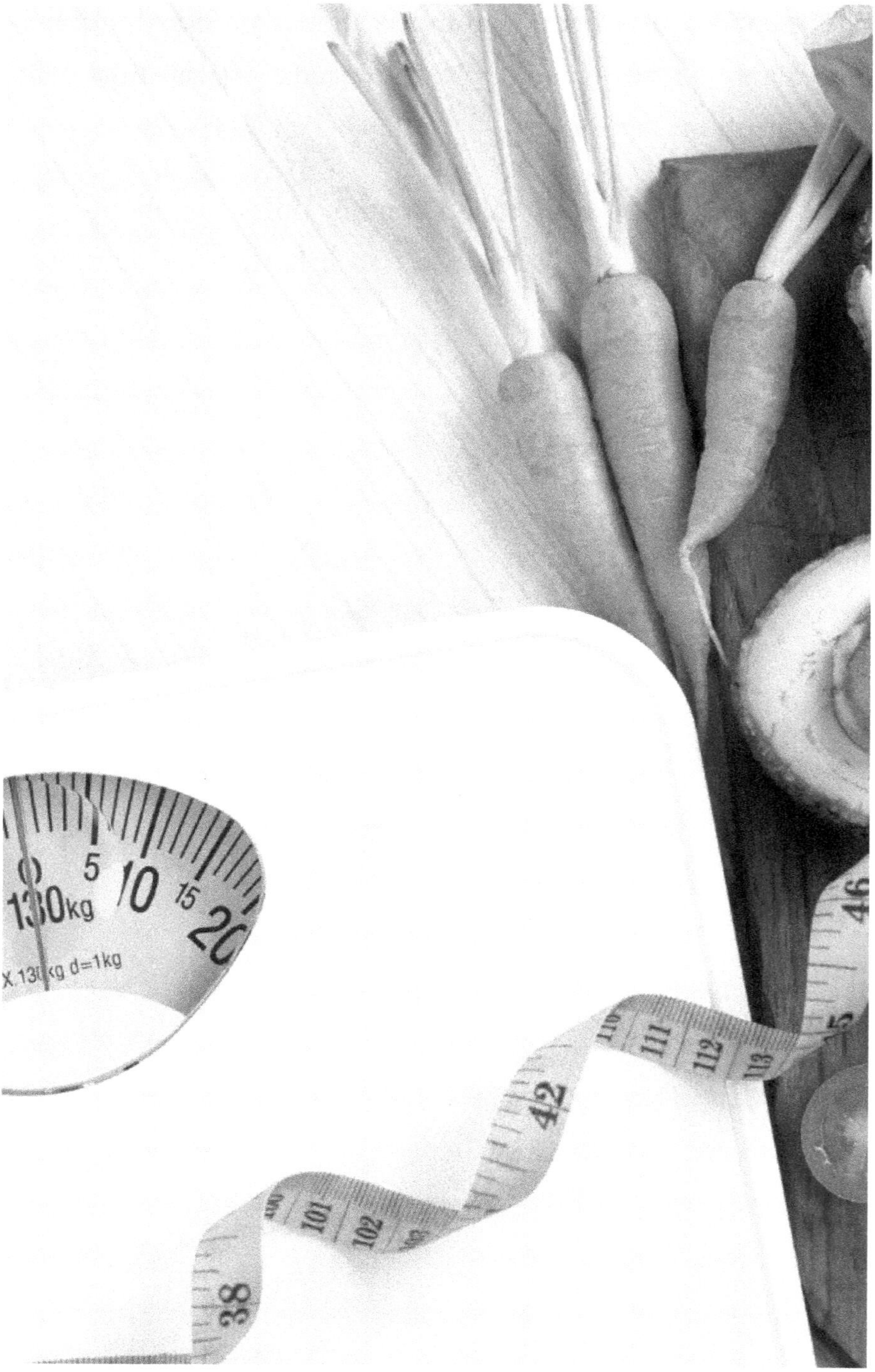
0 5 10 15 20
kg
d=1kg
101 102
42
111 112 113
38
46

Chapter 2.
Self-Hypnosis:
How It Works

O ne might ask, "How does hypnosis work?" the solution to the present question isn't definite. The mind has been an enormous puzzle among scientists, and a particular psychological state called Hypnosis may be a puzzle also. The only things that can be said about Hypnosis are the very things that happen in the hypnotic state. These are the behavioral changes and brain activities that a subject undergoes under Hypnosis. What remains a mystery for those who have studied Hypnosis 200 years ago can still be safely said.

What's Hypnosis?

The term "hypnosis" can be best described as an interaction between two people. If one of the people is trying to influence other people's perceptions, feelings, thinking, and behavior, then the former is called "hypnotist" and the latter the "subject." In this interaction, the hypnotist will ask the subject to concentrate on ideas and images that may evoke the intended responses. The verbal communications that the hypnotist uses to achieve these responses are named "hypnotic suggestions." If a person practiced the hypnotic procedures on his own without the help of a hypnotist, that activity is called "self-hypnosis."

How Self-Hypnosis Works

Performing self-spellbinding is as basic as having the option to move into a perspective that you are in when you are dreaming and resting.

The conscious mind in this state is relaxed, and your thoughts can flow freely to and from the subconscious.

Self-hypnosis for weight loss is a straightforward process, and it can be very relaxing as well. Self-hypnosis is all about getting in touch with our subconscious mind or body and talking to it or suggesting it.

Doing this can assist us with a wide range of things. Not exclusively will it assist us with accelerating our weight reduction, however, it can likewise help with sorrow, mending wounds, expanding confidence, assembling a superior body, recuperating inner wounds, or relieving maladies, and lots more.

> ➢ The process is very easy to perform; to begin, locate a decent calm spot to plunk down, don't rest since you

could nod off, and we don't need that to occur. Self-spellbinding for weight reduction can be unwinding and can make us nod off on the off chance that we are not cautious. We will likely have the option to speak with our inner mind. If we are dozing, at that point, this won't occur.

➤ So when you are plunking down in an agreeable position, you can be perched on a seat if this feels the most agreeable or on the floor, the best position is one where you are leaning against a divider with your legs loosened up before you.

➤ This position permits you to keep your back straight and feel the vitality stream from your toes to your head, sitting on a seat will help this too. In any case, the progression of vitality will be to some degree limited due to the bowed knees.

➤ After you are in your agreeable position, loosen up the entirety of your appendages, and take three full breaths. This causes us to unwind and prepare for our excursion into ourselves. Next, start by taking a gander at your toes and envision they are loose. Envision you can see vitality moving upwards from your toes toward your legs.

➤ Now look at your legs and feel them becoming completely relaxed, let them lay on the bed or against your chair, relax your shoulders and let your head rest nicely on your shoulders, feel your fingers all relaxed and feel the energy flowing from them and feel your arms completely relaxed.

➢ Now tell yourself out loud, you will walk down a flight of stairs to the count of 10; each time you count, take a step down. When you reach the last step, you will be in contact with your subconscious mind.

➢ Tell yourself this and then close your eyes and slowly count quietly, imagine a flight of stairs going down into a dark room, as you count to 10 each step starts to feel more substantial and you feel more relaxed when you reach the bottom step you should be in a state of self-hypnosis. This is where self-hypnosis for weight loss starts to work.

➢ Start by telling yourself that you are thin, lose 30 pounds, or 50 pounds, make it seem reasonable, tell yourself you look like an image you want to look like, then when you have finished, tell yourself you are going to walk back up the stairs. When you reach the top step at the count of 10, you will be fully awake.

Doing this self-hypnosis for weight loss exercise every day will help reprogram your subconscious mind to help you out with your weight loss.

You will lose weight much faster; it is also a great way to relax after a stressful day.

How to Change Your Thoughts

In the relaxed, attentive state of self-hypnosis, you can be more aware of what are usually "automatic" thoughts. One approach is to use one session to notice and remember the automatic thoughts that come up around a particular issue and then write down the thoughts and counter-thoughts you would like to replace them with.

For example, if one of your automatic thoughts was "I never succeed at anything," a counter-thought might be "I succeed at things often. When I do, I pay attention to them and congratulate myself."

Then, in a second session, you can practice saying the pair of thoughts, and gradually shifting the weight of credibility and commitment to the counter-thought.

How to Change Your Feelings

Changing emotions is very feasible with self-hypnosis. A straightforward technique is to connect with the feeling, give it a name (such as "anxiety"), and then notice how it feels in your body. Imagine what color it would be if it had a color, what texture it would have if it had a texture, what sound it might make. Then imagine that color, texture, or sound changing to one that is more pleasant.

Another emotional technique is to imagine your negative feeling on one hand and a positive feeling you want to replace it with on the other hand. Focus attention on them alternately, gradually bring them together and allow the positive attitude to be dominant as you close your hands together.

How to Change Your Behavior

In self-hypnosis, you can also visualize your future behavior as being different from what you would currently do in a particular set of circumstances. This mental pre-rehearsal or "future pacing" helps to prepare your mind to behave in that way in real life.

You can also motivate yourself by picturing the positive consequences of changing and comparing them with the negative consequences of staying the same.

How to Achieve Your Dreams

If you're clear in your mind about your dreams, you'll have some idea about the thoughts, feelings, and behaviors that belong to someone who's fulfilled those dreams. When you use self-hypnosis to move closer to being that kind of person, your dreams come closer to your grasp.

Emotional Side of Weight Loss and Why It's So Important

Calories in ought to be less than calories out - this is frequently affirmed to be the clear and successful equation of weight reduction.

The issue is that the technique doesn't work for some individuals. A solitary explanation exists for that reality - this recipe doesn't factor the passionate parts of getting in shape.

For some individuals, shedding pounds is a major battle. It incorporates longings, passionate eating, and addictions to specific nourishments.

These parts make it inconceivably hard to adequately present change and keep up a person's degree of joy and fulfillment.

Is it true that you are battling with your weight reduction goals? You aren't the only one!

A few elements could add to your disappointment, and disregarding the enthusiastic parts of weight addition and misfortune could likewise cause your issues.

The Most Powerful Emotional Components

Several emotional responses could interfere with losing weight and maintenance efforts. The most important ones include:

Anxiety and nervousness: for a few people, these feelings cause enthusiastic eating. When feeling apprehensive, these people need an outlet and a wellspring of solace. Food is much of the time this outlet. Food "perks up" these people and empowers them to keep working while at the same time holding the adverse feelings within proper limits.

Exercise phobia: a passionate component that is regularly thought little of. Numerous individuals accept that activity is unimaginably unpleasant. Some stress over getting to the rec center because of their present weight.They lack motivation, never enjoyed sports, and believe that the situation isn't going to be much different this time around.

Body image: how do you perceive yourself? The lack of confidence and love for yourself could prevent you from getting to that ideal weight. You may think that you simply don't deserve change or aren't ok to possess a healthy and fit body. This is why you're probably sabotaging your weight loss efforts.

Previously mentioned are not many of the normal intense subject matters remaining inside the method of fruitful weight reduction. For certain individuals, it could be much increasingly convoluted. An awful connection with food, compulsion, and reliance is a significantly increasingly genuine mental issue that makes weight reduction unimaginable.

How to affect the Emotional Aspect of Weight Loss

Dealing with emotions should happen before you modify your diet or start understanding. You need to be motivated, and you can't do that if you aren't in the right state of mind. Weight loss hypnosis may be a good option for accomplishing that change.

Through hypnotherapy for weight loss, you'll get to identify why you don't have the confidence or why you've established a destructive relationship with food. The process is far from stressful. It will offer you more power and control than trying to face those negative emotions on your own.

Weight loss hypnosis works on a subconscious level. Thus, through the assistance of a therapist, you'll easily replace the destructive thought patterns with far more productive "mantras." once you complete the hypnotherapy for weight loss process, you'll find it much easier to enjoy healthy foods, feel excited about exercising, and start accepting your body.

Weight reduction is intricate, though masters attempt to push their "straightforward" equations. For a beginning, you have to comprehend the feelings that disrupt the general flow of accomplishment. When you address these negative thoughts,you'll find it easier to get started on a healthier and happier journey.

Then Why Do People Fear Hypnosis?

Something that causes individuals to delay utilizing a trance inducer or to utilize self-mesmerizing is that they imagine that entrancing is risky.

Indeed, in all cases, the response to this inquiry is that mesmerizing isn't risky. Part of what people seek once they are looking to use a hypnotist is to seek someone who will make them do something they cannot do or don't want to do.

Furthermore, this idea that they could have this sort of relationship with someone else likewise frightens them. All things considered, the trance inducer can't transform you into a reluctant member in anything! The trance inducer can just help you with what you're willing and prepared to achieve.

Working with a hypnotist will help you see, feel, and act fully congruent with what you really want to accomplish. There's no danger in seeking the assistance of a hypnotist or using self-hypnosis techniques to help you briefly or future goals.

As you weigh the dangers of remaining the same, doing the same unhealthy behaviors day in and day out, you can see that they certainly outweigh any mythical dangers you thought you would experience from hypnosis or self-hypnosis because there is no greater joy than being in control of your destiny.

The Key to Making Self-Hypnosis Work

Self-hypnosis has been employed by an excellent many of us to make real, measurable changes in themselves and their lives. Immense quantities of individuals have used the office of self-spellbinding to dispense with fears, control torment, treat physical and mental manifestations, as well as utilizing it to prevail in their objectives.

Notwithstanding, numerous others have accomplished nothing advantageous from its utilization despite the fact that specialists state that everybody is hypnotizable! All in all, the inquiry remains - Why doesn't it generally work?

Many people fail to achieve any measurable results from self-hypnosis because they're not using it correctly!

The initial step you should take when considering utilizing self-entrancing is to comprehend what you might want. Despite the fact that this may sound rudimentary and a bit of deigning, truly think about it. Do you know correctly, directly down to the last detail, what you might want to acknowledge from your self-spellbinding project?Or, do you listen to a generic self-hypnosis session and hope for the best?

For example, taking note of a self-hypnosis recording for more confidence could also be an honest goal, but how does one quantify confidence?

Do you want to be confident around people or potential mates? It is sheltered to state that you are attempting to recognize more trust in your movement or work-life? Is it actually that you need to be progressively sure about your capacities, and in this way, it is your confidence that you wish to construct?

For self-hypnosis, like all other self-improvement techniques, to be effective, you want to use it with a goal in mind! Your objective, to be utilized with self-mesmerizing, must be exact.

Take a stab at recording a rundown of things you might want to accomplish and afterward organize them. Take your most fundamental want and switch it into an objective. Might you be able to record it? Kindly do it now!

Have you done it?

By recording your objective, you transform it into an aim - a goal that can be acknowledged through the intensity of self-mesmerizing.

This makes your craving genuine and substantial and not an obscure wish or dream. By doing this, you have recently made a solid self-spellbinding objective!

Since you are sure about what you need and have made your first self-mesmerizing objective, you have to complete this fundamental work before entering a self-entrancing state.

You must now rewrite your goal in the present tense as though you already have it. Some people find they experience discomfort when they word a goal in the present tense because it feels too unreal.

On the off chance that this transpires, re-word the objective to mirror the way that it is occurring. Never express an objective later on tense! Never state what you are doing, not need or incorporate any of the things that you essentially attempt to wipe out!

Your self-hypnosis goal must state your intention positively and only include what you would like. "I am sans obligation" is an awful model, to be sans obligation, you should initially consider obligation! "I am prosperous and rich," is vastly improved as it incorporates what you do need! "I am not, at this point awkward in social circumstances," as awful as you are concentrating on your absence of certainty! "I am a highly confident one that is comfortable with others in any situation," is far more suitable because it states the positive outcome you're seeking!

The psyche mind works, not in words, but in pictures. This turns out to be evident during self-mesmerizing. So whatever you do well as of now, don't think about an elephant! What's your opinion of? An elephant! Isn't that so?

In order not to consider an elephant, your subconscious has got to produce an image of an elephant, so it knows what you do not want to think about! This is why it's crucial never to include what you do not want in your self-hypnosis goal!

As you enter a self-entrancing stupor and utilize this state to reinvent your brain, your psyche brain will normally frame pictures from the words you hear or use. So just utilize positive, objective insisting articulations! Guarantee your announcements are nitty-gritty, positive, and forthright. Doing this will drive your inner mind brains to make pictures that fortify your wants, and it will utilize them as a manual for making your future!

Weight Loss Self Hypnosis

In a supersized world, individuals have numerous chances to eat and drink WAY excessively, yet what's behind corpulence is normally more than longing for a huge request of fries.

In America, a genuine eating regimen industry has developed around obesity. It powers overweight individuals to follow through on a significant expense for in vogue diets, pills, or costly and high-hazard medical procedures. By doing away with starches or fat, taking pills or infusions, sprinkling gems on your food, falling back on careful medication, or drinking naturally-occurring diet elixirs, numerous health food nuts briefly lose pounds however, they don't lose the outlook which contributes to weight gain.

The outcome is that after such difficult work and conceivably burning through a huge number of dollars, most calorie counters recover their weight and feel significantly progressively disheartened.Weight loss hypnosis can assist you to change how you feel and get control of your bad dieting habits.

Hypnosis for Weight Loss - What Can Hypnosis Do?

Hypnosis may be defined as a routine inducing an alternate state of awareness, which helps persons become highly sensitive to a hypnotist's suggestions. This routine has been accepted in psychoanalysis for treating psychic illnesses by revisiting the harmful events which caused them in the past and then by transmitting suggestions created to assist them.

- **Hypnosis may be used to overcome phobias.** Hypnosis may be used to lessen stress or tension. Hypnosis may help you remain calm before a big test and during your big speech. You will most certainly benefit from Hypnosis.

- **Hypnosis may regulate blood flow and different autonomic functions** that are not generally subject to conscious manipulation. The relaxing reaction that occurs with Hypnosis also alters the Neuro-hormonal systems that regulate many body functions.

- **Hypnosis for weight loss may assist you in passing when everything else has failed.** Using Hypnosis, we may aid you to achieve the weight loss that you want. Hypnosis may go straight to the middle of the matter and specialize in replacing particular behavior or habits with healthy choices.

- **Hypnosis may also be used to transform those who are hurt by anxiety attacks.** These are characterized by the inability to concentrate, problems in making decisions, extreme sensitivity, disharmony, sleep interruptions, excessive sweating, and consistent muscle tension.

- **Hypnosis may aid by giving you coping systems so that you can face them in more appropriate ways whenever stress-inducing situations happen.** Hypnosis may be used in many various ways.

- **Hypnosis may also be a method of pain control,** often used with burn victims and women in labor. Hypnosis cannot depose an exercise outline but may implement and strengthen it.

- **Hypnotic affirmations have a cumulative therapeutic effect in the subconscious part of the mind,** with the capability of improving healthy self-esteem. Hypnosis can't make a person to do anything against their will or that contradicts their values.

- A Hypnotherapist has ethics that are required to create only those changes that abide by agreed-upon change work.

- **Hypnosis can help you obtain personal achievements and help you remain motivated toward obtaining those goals.** After a few sessions of "hypnosis therapy," you may find more willingness to live and have more energy than ever imagined.

Weight Loss Hypnosis Breaks Down WHY You Eat

Hypnosis training has assisted people to lose weight sustainably by changing how they feel about their eating, reducing pressure and stress, and relaxing. Overeating has nothing to do with hunger. Instead, it has everything to do with high stress, racing thoughts, and other negative emotional feelings that food allows a person to distract them from feeling.

Like all Hypnosis, weight reduction involvesthe utilization of the intensity of proposal while individuals are loose as long as the recommendations are reliable with what the individual WANTS to do in any case. Some portion of the accentuation is on moving inclinations and decisions toward better food decisions and conquering your food desires.

Since numerous health food nuts have negative idea designs that urge them to utilize doughnuts and mushy bacon bowls to shift how they feel, weight reduction mesmerizing additionally urges you to consider yourself to be a hearty one that needn't bother with food to differ anything. You figure out how to see changing eating designs not as hardship yet as engaging and simple since it's what you need to do in any case.

How to benefit from Hypnosis naturally

Since any such encouraging beliefs in our subconscious can have damaging effects on our lives, Hypnosis aims to change these beliefs positively. The manner in which it works is by the trancelike orders entering your brain, and focusing on the negative and restricting convictions that impact your life and your outcomes.

Spellbinding helps by unpretentiously affecting upon these convictions inside you. It changes your reasoning like those of an easily thin and sound individual. When you begin thinking along these lines, you also can get more fit impressively and normally while really keeping it off because of the change at the inner mind level.

What it would take for you is to be available to this incredibly ground-breaking, progressively mainstream, and demonstrated thought, checking out of it and getting a charge out of the outcomes.

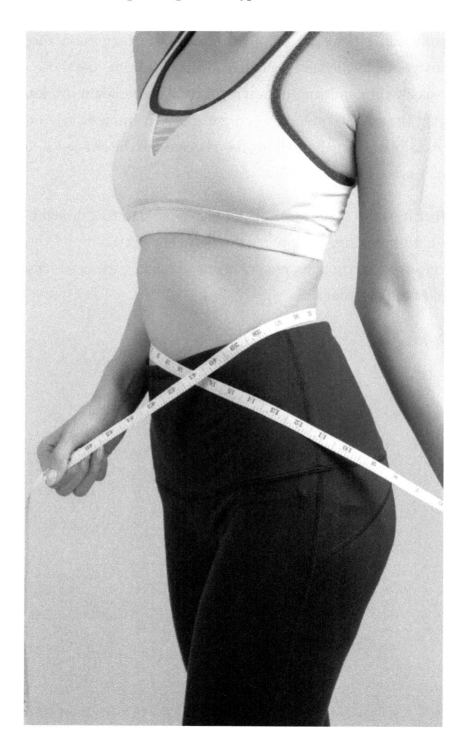

Chapter 3.
The Benefit of Hypnosis in Weight Loss

Ever since Hypnosis has been used for self-improvement, many people have managed to use Hypnosis for weight loss.

This method is really beneficial because once the sessions are over,the subconscious has been successfully rewritten; then, we can notice some unusual benefits, like a person would rather walk then drive without thinking about it consciously.

This and more positive lifestyle changes will follow when you use Hypnosis for weight loss.

Self-Hypnosis for Weight Loss

Over many decades, people have tried almost every possible way to lose those extra pounds.

If you're one of those that have tried everything and zip seems to figure, then there's another exciting option. Have you ever tried self-hypnosis for weight loss?

Self-hypnosis has worked for several people, but unfortunately, it doesn't work for everybody. In saying this, self-hypnosis for weight loss features a high enough success rate to form a viable weight-loss strategy.

As intriguing as this sounds; there are two sides to this method that you should be aware of. Let's take a gaze at the pros of using self-hypnosis for weight loss.

Pro: Self-Hypnosis does not require special equipment.

The obvious one is that as you're doing the Hypnosis yourself, you will not need a hypnotist! Unlike most weight loss programs, self-hypnosis requires nothing more but you and your belief.

However, it's advisable if this is your first time at self-hypnosis for weight loss, that you simply visit a hypnotherapist so as to become conversant with the method.

If you are also new to diet and exercise, the benefits far outweigh the cost of consulting a doctor and a nutritionist to put together a healthy eating and exercise plan that's right for you. Combined with the self-hypnosis for the weight-loss method, you are on the right path to slimming down at an accelerated rate.

Pro: Self-hypnosis is an established self-help mechanism

Throughout the years, Hypnosis has been utilized to help in the recuperation of lost recollections and to assist individuals with kicking the propensity for smoking.Fans swear by it, but many people are still very skeptical of its merits. Regardless of whether you're a fan or a skeptic, one thing is certain: Self-hypnosis has helped thousands of people lose weight and will continue to help thousands more.

Although it's not really understood why self-hypnosis for weight loss works if you speak to someone who has used self-hypnosis to reduce, you'll likely be told that it worked for them after everything else failed. Such stories are still common, even to the present day.

If you've used other weight loss methods previously and that they haven't worked for you, you would possibly want to offer self-hypnosis a try. It's harmless, and you never know - it just might work!

Hypnosis and Self-Hypnosis for Weight Loss

The idea of utilizing Hypnosis or self-spellbinding for weight reduction is interesting, and it is ideal to have faith in, yet is it without a doubt? The thought isn't exactly as unrealistic as it used to be, since today, more individuals know about how the inner mind functions. Spellbinding and self-mesmerizing are presently utilized for an assortment of purposes. While not yet precisely standard, the thought is, in any event, acknowledged as conceivable by many.

Carefully, nobody is stating that you can't cause pounds to vanish by Hypnosis, like by enchantment. No, Hypnosis is intended to reinvent your inner mind with the goal that you carry on in an unexpected way. All things considered, your activities have a great deal to do with your weight, just as numerous different parts of your physical wellbeing. Put that way; it doesn't appear to be so difficult to accept.

So what sort of changes would hypnosis be able to cause in our conduct?

- Eat Less - devour less calories

- Eat Healthier - settle on better decisions when shopping/cooking/requesting out

- Exercise More - more inspiration when working out

- Improved Self Image - decrease self-damage

Would hypnosis be able to do every one of these things? Hypothetically, yes. Accomplishes it generally works this well for each and every individual who attempts it? Tragically, No. Nothing works for everyone, including diets, exercise, or diet pills.

Utilizing Hypnosis for Weight Loss

In the event that you needed to shed pounds utilizing Hypnosis, how might you go about it? All things considered, you could visit a certified trance specialist. While this wouldn't be modest, contrasted with any conventional treatment, it has the upside of being quick-acting. Most trance specialists center around showing you strategies you can use all alone, so you don't need to come back to them for meetings continually.

Another alternative is to discover one of the numerous accounts that are intended to assist you with getting thinner. These can be played whenever it might suit you, however, you can't play them while driving or doing anything where your full conscious consideration is required.

One Tool among Many

Try not to anticipate that Hypnosis should work without anyone else. Obviously, the general purpose is that it should make it simpler for you to adhere to your eating regimen, practice program, and different objectives. In any case, your conscious psyche needs to help it along by trying your best to remain focused.

Since Hypnosis centers on your psyche, it's despite everything up to you to locate the outside apparatuses that work best for you.

As it were, you ought to do your findings and locate a sound eating regimen that concurs with your body (not all weight control plans function admirably for each individual).

The same is valid for a workout. If you don't like setting off to the rec center, you shouldn't attempt to entrance yourself into adoring it. Work with your common inclinations, and get yourself to practice such that is reliable with your inclinations.

The genuine target of Hypnosis for weight reduction is to permit you to do the things you need to never really weight without applying so much self-control. On the off chance that your psyche mind is more in agreement with your fitness objectives, there's to a lesser extent an opportunity that you'll attack yourself by undermining your eating routine or forsaking your activity program.

Utilizing Hypnosis to get thinner may sound bizarre or extraordinary. However, it's simply one more approach to utilize your brain to help your objectives. It may not be for everybody, except if the thought sounds engaging or fascinating, you might need to investigate a portion of the opportunities for getting in shape utilizing Hypnosis.

If you take a gander at the 10,000foot view, Hypnosis would be beneficial for you regardless of whether you didn't lose any weight. Try not to stress; if you do attempt Hypnosis for weight reduction, you will get in shape.

One thing that you just need to bear in mind is Hypnosis for weight reduction is certainly not an enchantment pill. You will in any case need to need to get thinner, and it will even now take a portion of your determination. You have to follow the Hypnosis for the health improvement plan you pick and stick with it. If you do these straightforward things, you can be headed to a more joyful, slimmer you.

Weight Loss through Hypnosis: Myth or Fact?

Weight loss through hypnosis, is that a fact? Is that just a bunch of well-placed lies? Are people really going to believe that you can actually eliminate fat from your body through a process as controversial as hypnosis? Well, believe it or not, several studies prove the efficiency and honesty of this method.

While weight loss through hypnosis might not work for every single person in the world, it's certainly worth your time as it has helped thousands before.

You see, hypnosis is all about disposition. If you can change someone's disposition into doing something (or stop doing it for that matter), you will eventually change the way they live, right?

That is a fact, and hypnosis is that practice with which you can change the way someone acts or even thinks. And here is where weight loss through hypnosis comes into play; it is not that hard to switch someone's thoughts into being someone healthier. Since hypnosis is focused directly into someone's subconscious, it is quite easy to program their weight loss behavior.

Lose Weight With Hypnosis - Myth Or Fact?

"Overeating" and "overweight" are directly related, right?

There a variety of reasons a person would overeat. It may be an emotional attachment to food, maybe just emotional eating to cope, maybe plain old bad eating habits, or we try every fad diet out there, end up quitting and gaining more weight than we originally had to lose in the first place.

Whatever the reason, lose weight by hypnosis strategies can help most anyone overcome their issues. You know that if you eat less and exercise more, the pounds would just come off, right?

But it's not that easy...

There is so much going on in our minds, conscious and subconscious!

We may make a conscious decision to lose weight, but our subconscious is not on board for unknown reasons. Using a loose weight/hypnosis package from a credible source, a person can access his/her subconscious mind, find out what issues are holding him/her back, and rewrite the program in their mind. The subconscious mind is where all of our bad habits, emotional issues, and food attachments are found.

However, this process only works with people who are actually willing to be hypnotized. There are plenty of people out there with which hypnosis is utterly inefficient, mainly because of the way they think and the impermeability of their ideals and beliefs. If you are one such person, then weight loss through hypnosis will be an outstanding failure.

Still, if you are open to new ideas and solutions, then your mind might be susceptible to hypnosis. Therefore you could start losing incredible amounts of weight after being hypnotized.

Keep in mind that weight loss through hypnosis expands into many different areas for attacking the problem, it's not that you will miraculously lose this weight, it rather means that you are going to desire to follow a weight loss plan truly and that your willpower will be severely enhanced, allowing you to stay inside your weight loss path without feeling the urge to drop out.

It is additionally very important to take note of that, if you choose to finish a weight loss trance program, you see all the outcomes this may include.You will be allowing an outsider into the very depths of your mind. You will permit him to reprogram the very concepts of life that you have constructed in your lifetime.

This doesn't necessarily mean anything bad, but you must note that before attempting to sign up to a weight loss through hypnosis program.

The Benefits of Learning Self-Hypnosis Techniques

Hypnosis is a representation of what is within you, your strengths, and yourcapabilities. Narrowing and focusing your intense concentration and a spotlight on something that you simply want to vary. It is mind over matter.

You are releasing the complete potential and capability of your mind to draw in positive energy. Learning self-hypnosis techniques offers a lot of benefits. Hypnosis can be used to change something about yourself that will make you more productive, happier, and a better person.

Rapid Weight Loss Hypnosis for Women

People have the wrong notion about Hypnosis, maybe because of what they have seen in movies. You don't have to be in a spell or trance to be in Hypnosis. Many of our daily activities are performed under Hypnosis without us being conscious about it.

Driving a car, for instance, is one of them. It is an activity that you shut your mind out of other stimuli or distractions to concentrate on driving. Your concentration and focus will help you to respond to anything that will happen while driving automatically.

The benefits of learning self-hypnosis techniques:

❖ **Change Yourself.** Learning self-hypnosis techniques will help you change your negative thinking into a positive attitude. You can even learn how to control anger through Hypnosis. It can assist you to improve your self-confidence and overcome shyness and fears. Learning self-hypnosis techniques will allow you to relax and focus on something that you want to enhance and change. Hypnosis will also allow you to overcome challenging situations in your life.

❖ **Overcome Diseases.** Clinical Hypnosis is officially recognized by the American Medical Association and, therefore, the American Psychological Association. Learning self-hypnosis techniques can help you overcome diseases and pains. There are self-hypnosis techniques that you can use to conquer migraines, insomnia, menstrual pains, anxiety, panic attacks, and even overcome fears of dental procedures.

❖ **Weight loss.** Learning self-hypnosis techniques also will assist you to stop over-eating to scale back weight. It will help you gain your ideal weight without feeling deprived or hungry. The mind is in charge of metabolism, and in changing your mind, you can change metabolism. You will learn to stop compulsive eating, take charge of your weight, and shed off those unwanted fats.

❖ **Quit bad habits and addiction.** Another benefit of learning self-hypnosis techniques is the capability to quit bad habits and addiction like smoking and drinking alcohol. Hypnosis is being used now as a smoking cessation therapy. Learning self-hypnosis techniques will help you deal with the psychological and emotional phase of giving up smoking.

❖ **Enhance Relationships.** Hypnosis can do wonders for your relationship and sexual love. You can achieve dating success and attract the love you deserve.

Learning self-hypnosis techniques will allow you to program yourself for unstoppable confidence to make positive changes in your dating life.

If you are interested in learning self-hypnosis techniques, it is recommended that you get advice from a certified Clinical Hypnotherapist.

Hypnosis isn't the sole cure for all of your problems. Still, it is a good alternative that many people find effective.

Benefits of Hypnosis for Weight Loss

Weight loss can require tremendous effort, especially if you've chosen the incorrect approach. The probabilities are that you've got tried a minimum of several different methodologies, which you've discovered that each one of them is ineffective.

Many weight loss methods fail because they provide only a partial solution.

A comprehensive approach is one that will producea long-term and sustainable advantage. Weight loss hypnosis is one such methodology.

Is it true that you are asking why hypnotherapy for weight reduction is more proficient than prohibitive systems?

Several benefits of the effectiveness of using Hypnosis for weight loss

People typically have one of three reactions upon hearing the word hypnosis. One, they may be cynical and think they don't need to look any further into the whole process. Second, they may think this is a risky procedure.

If this is the case, they will be hesitant to use Hypnosis for any reason. Finally, some will be curious and look more into what Hypnosis is and how it works. It is easy to have doubts about a subject you know little or nothing about. By learning about

Hypnosis for weight loss, you can find the truth and benefit yourself.

Hypnosis is a dream state in which you are focused on a particular area. It is very similar to REM (rapid eye movement) sleep, which is an important part of rejuvenating your body. Most people don't have problems going to sleep at night. Once you realize that Hypnosis is a slightly different form of essential sleep, you can relax and feel positive that you are not being controlled by someone else.

While hypnotized, you still can think logically. Other portions of your mind are just more open to change. You are in control at all times. The hypnotist is just there to help you. A hypnotist must be flexible and adaptable to be effective. Each subject is different, so each hypnosis session must also be unique.

Hypnosis is not a form of activity. It is a life-changing procedure that works with most people. Heroin addicts can get off of the drugs and stay off of them. Hypnosis for weight loss will keep the pounds off for good.

This technique can change your life for the better in so many ways. If you have an area that you are struggling with and conquer it with the help of Hypnosis, you will also gain confidence in other areas. Your entire life can change as a result of successful Hypnosis.

Hypnosis is a great learning tool that can be used by almost any human being. A slightly different form of Hypnosis is used every time you focus on something and give it your undivided attention.

You need to be comfortable with Hypnosis for it to work. Think of it as your friend.

Hypnosis is a natural process that many use daily. You often don't even know they are doing so. Anyone can become skilled at and benefit from this technique, and you do not have to worry about side effects. There are none with this behavior modification method.

Whether you are looking into Hypnosis for weight loss or fear of flying, you can succeed. **Hypnosis allows you to try new things in a controlled environment.** You can practice new behaviors before actually engaging in them. If you are looking to get control over your behavior and your life in general, give Hypnosis a try. You have nothing to fear, as this is a natural process that provides instant results.

You don't have to worry about negative consequences, and self-hypnosis can be practiced anywhere. You will grow as a human being, and the results will be astounding.

Hypnosis Helps in Breaking the Addiction. A few people have a profoundly unfortunate relationship with food. It gives comfort that no other movement is fit for conveying. Food is not any longer viewed as a sort of nourishment; it becomes a coping mechanism.

The more you eat, the higher you are feeling. This is often why you continue eating even after you've reached the purpose of satiety.

Weight loss hypnotherapy is often wont to break the addictive nature of this coping mechanism. An experienced therapist can change the connection with food and replace it with a healthier coping mechanism. Such habits are often introduced on a subconscious level, making the transition easier one.

You can put into practice Self-Hypnosis for Weight Loss from the comfort of your house.

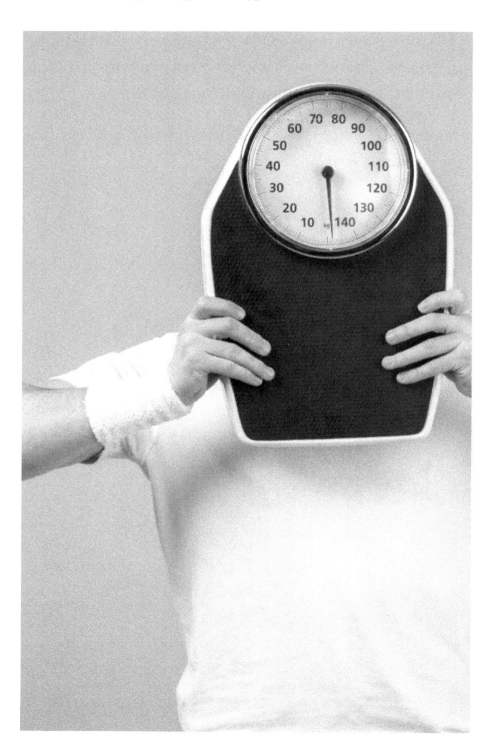

Chapter 4.
Weight Loss Hypnosis Routine and How to Practice It Every Day

It is not always easy to lose weight when our eating habits have been established for years: need a little sweetness in the morning, ice cream in the evening in front of our favorite series... Hypnosis offers to help us get rid of our bad reflexes.

What is Hypnosis?

How does it work?

Can you lose weight with Hypnosis?

To accomplish your ideal load without yielding your everyday way of life and wellbeing practice, in this part, we will have a discussion on the training for an exceptionally viable hypnosis Weight Loss Plan.

These practices and schedules are profoundly required to adjust your body against weight gain, which will assist you with learning the genuine pith of getting in shape normally.

Here is a definitive rundown of Practices for profoundly powerful spellbinding weight-reduction plan:

Hypnotic Practices to Help You Take Off Pounds

As time goes on, there are more and more reports of dieters using Hypnosis to achieve significant weight loss. Isn't it gratifying to read about actual cases where people are now enjoying a slimmer and healthier body through Hypnosis?

It is true; Hypnosis can help even the most weak-willed among us to shed some unwanted pounds. And it does this by helping us change our thought process. Indeed, hypnotic weight loss techniques help us to require healthy foods over the junk that we usually crave.

Here are the top hypnotic suggestions:
✓ **Stop Sugar Hypnosis**

The suggestion is planted that sugar is not that exciting. Once this idea is in place, your body will benefit in many ways. In addition to weight loss, the hypnotic dieter will experience better concentration, deeper sleeping patterns, and a much-improved quality of life.

✓ Comfort eating is a bad idea.

How frequently have you sat down, baffled, frantic, bothered, discouraged, or desolate, winding up going after a sack of potato chips, a bunch of treats, that half-gallon of frozen yogurt, or another food to help facilitate the issue.

Solace eating is a colossal issue for some individuals who discover impermanent delight in a pack of potato chips, a gallon of frozen yogurt, or a sheet of treats.Hypnosis can easily work its magic on the subconscious mind to give the dieter more control over what they put in their mouth.

✓ Fast food is really bad.

It doesn't need any scientist to figure out that fast foods are to be avoided. They're loaded with fat and high carbohydrates, which translate to clogged arteries and unwanted pounds.

Now, what if you may perhaps use Hypnosis to eliminate your fast food desires? Hypnosis gives you control over fast food impulses, which means you end up choosing healthy alternatives.

✓ Chocolate is to be avoided.

If you're like me, you find the chocolate's cravings to be among the hardest to eradicate. Hypnosis can supply a much-needed enhance to your subconscious mind and help you get your priorities in place. It can actually convince you that you have no interest in eating chocolate!

✓ Healthy eating Hypnosis

Have you noticed that as soon as you stop working for a few days, you immediately have a tendency to addmore weight? This is because you continue to eat without burning as many calories. Playing sports only increases appetite, but does not perk up assimilation.

By rehearsing yoga and reflection, absorption improves, and the craving for fatty food diminishes. So you are eager, however, your craving is happy with lesser amounts.This has a long term effect on weight. Even if you can't exercise for a few days, you're not going to start gaining weight all of a sudden.

✓ Emotional eating hypnosis

The next time you stuff yourself with chocolate or some other kind of junk food, watch for a while: why do you do this? Are you stressed for any reason (at work or at home)? Stress has a direct impact on the tendency to snack from time to time.

This temporarily relieves stress. However, when you meditate, you naturally release the stress that is deeply embedded in the system. It is a healthier way to combat stress and also to be in good shape.

✓ Regular exercise

The standard exercise program isn't unfamiliar to us, yet the issue is discipline. In the event that you are not intellectually arranged to do a wellness movement consistently, you not, slim or lose those extra knots on your gut. Exercise comes in various structures, and that is the thing that makes this propensity a great one.

Any physical activities, for instance, moving, sports, swimming, walking, running, cycling, or even your standard morning vehicle wash would all have the option to add to your action plan.So are you tired of having a regular exercise? You decide!

✓ A daily dose of meditation

Meditation is a practice that helps relax the mind and body with powerful techniques. Once you focus on meditation, you also apply a good posture that constitutes a fine body figure.

Integrating mindfulness as one of your weight loss plans is a sure way to lose weight without too much stress and financial expenditures naturally. Truly, meditation is one sole practice that can give you health and wellness and Lose Weight potentials.

✓ **Stop Junk Food Hypnosis**

Instead of receiving a lessening diet, just change the manner in which you eat. Eat four to six little dinners for the duration of the day to keep your digestion dynamic. Evade greasy nourishments, eat sugars with some restraint, and eat a lot of new products of the soil.

Maintain a strategic distance from handled nourishments to bring down your sodium admission. An excessive amount of sodium can trigger water weight and moderate your weight reduction endeavors.

✓ **Avoid terrible ways of life**

Ways of life can either have negative or constructive outcomes on our body, contingent in certainty upon your picked propensities. Terrible ways of life, similar to overconsumption of liquor drinks, smoking, illicit medication use, and bunches of others, will unavoidably make your wellbeing debase and create infections.

What is more terrible is that it could prompt weight as an excessive amount of liquor gives a high centralization of calories, particularly lager. So whether you're on a weight-reduction plan or not, avoid those awful indecencies to deal with constitution and appropriate weight.

✓ Be sociable and have fun

Did you know that a sociable person is more immune to weight gain? Are you probably wondering how? The research concludes that being fun and sociable can develop the so-called "brown fats" that help lessen the white fats in the body.

White fat establishes to weight gain while earthy colored fat is normally found in babies. Through sociable interaction, brown fats can be developed and will add as your friendly Lose Weight buddy.

✓ Control your cravings

This is one inclination that you ought to effectively apply to your weight-reduction plan. The whole way across our environmental factors, various enticements can draw us out of our weight-reduction plan. There are sweet nourishments, lousy nourishments, prepared food sources, and numerous different items that can at last signify our weight.

Applying an exacting control can give us the best possible course for weight reduction achievement. Drive your psyche the correct way, and you will positively forestall weight gain.

These practices for highly effective hypnosis weight loss can help you out of your weight gain dilemma. Keeping a healthy lifestyle and a trusted weight loss habit can overcome any weight-loss issue.

How to Self-Hypnotize for Weight Loss

The procedure of Hypnosis is getting your psyche into a state where it can acknowledge a proposal. During Hypnosis, a subject can bring an excursion profound into their inner mind to dispense with convictions and propensities that might be hindering to his regular daily existence.

This is the reason Hypnosis is so well known for those trying to lessen. In any case, it isn't imperative to look for and pay for a specialist. Most protection plans don't take care of the cost of hypnotherapy too. Attempt to self-entrance yourself to lose additional weight.

Stage 1

Schedule time in your day where you won't be sidetracked by outer activities. Attempt to set aside at least half-hour where you'll inundate yourself during a daze. It is imperative to concentrate during this whole timeframe.

Stage 2

Set weight reduction objectives for yourself. Focus on a precise measure of weight you need to lose and a particular time you need to lose it. Peruse this objective out loud before you start.

Stage 3

Envision yourself as the size you necessitate to be. Envision what your body will resemble once you achieve your optimal weight. Also, consider how others will respond and what they will say. Attempt to make the scene as distinctive as conceivable rich with shading, scents, sounds, and emotions.

Stage 4

Close your eyes, and relax up your body until it is totally limp. Contribute in profound relaxation for 3 minutes until you feel an impression from your skull to your feet. After the sensation is felt, loosen up that piece of your body. You will be in a stupor state.

Stage 5

Envision your optimal self in a stupor state. Consider how you will see the world, how others will see you, and how great it will feel to be solid and fit as a swindle. Take a gander at your body in its fit, trim state.

Stage 6

Return to your current state gradually. Be certain you bring the sentiments of the inner experience back with you. Doing this day by day will prepare your brain to feel how great it will be to shed pounds. You will step by step build the conduct alterations important to get in shape.

Self-Hypnosis: How Do We Do It?

Self-hypnosis takes up the rules and techniques of classic Hypnosis, with the difference that the hypnotherapist is yourself.

The Preparation

It is recommended, practicing self-hypnosis while sitting on a comfortable armchair or sofa, feet flat on the floor, and hands on your thighs. All in complete silence, of course: you turn off your laptop and the TV!

Then we close our eyes and create a vacuum. This moment is close to meditation: it is a matter of becoming aware of each part of your body, starting from the feet and gradually going up to the head, breathing deeply.

It is only once completely relaxed that we can begin the self-suggestion phase.

Self-Suggestion

First, rule number 1 of self-hypnosis (and Hypnosis) is to treat only one problem at a time. If you suffer from both anxiety and lack of self-confidence, you devote a separate session to each of these problems.

Once the problem has been identified, we mentally address the unconscious to guide it toward resolving this problem.

This is where rule number 2 comes in: self-hypnosis is self-suggestion. It should not be a set of self-imposed orders. Sentences must always be positive. For example, we don't say, "you shouldn't be afraid," but "I'm not afraid anymore."

Also, we favor positive terms: better to say, "I know I will succeed" rather than "I no longer know failure" because failure is a strong and negative word on which the unconscious can focus.

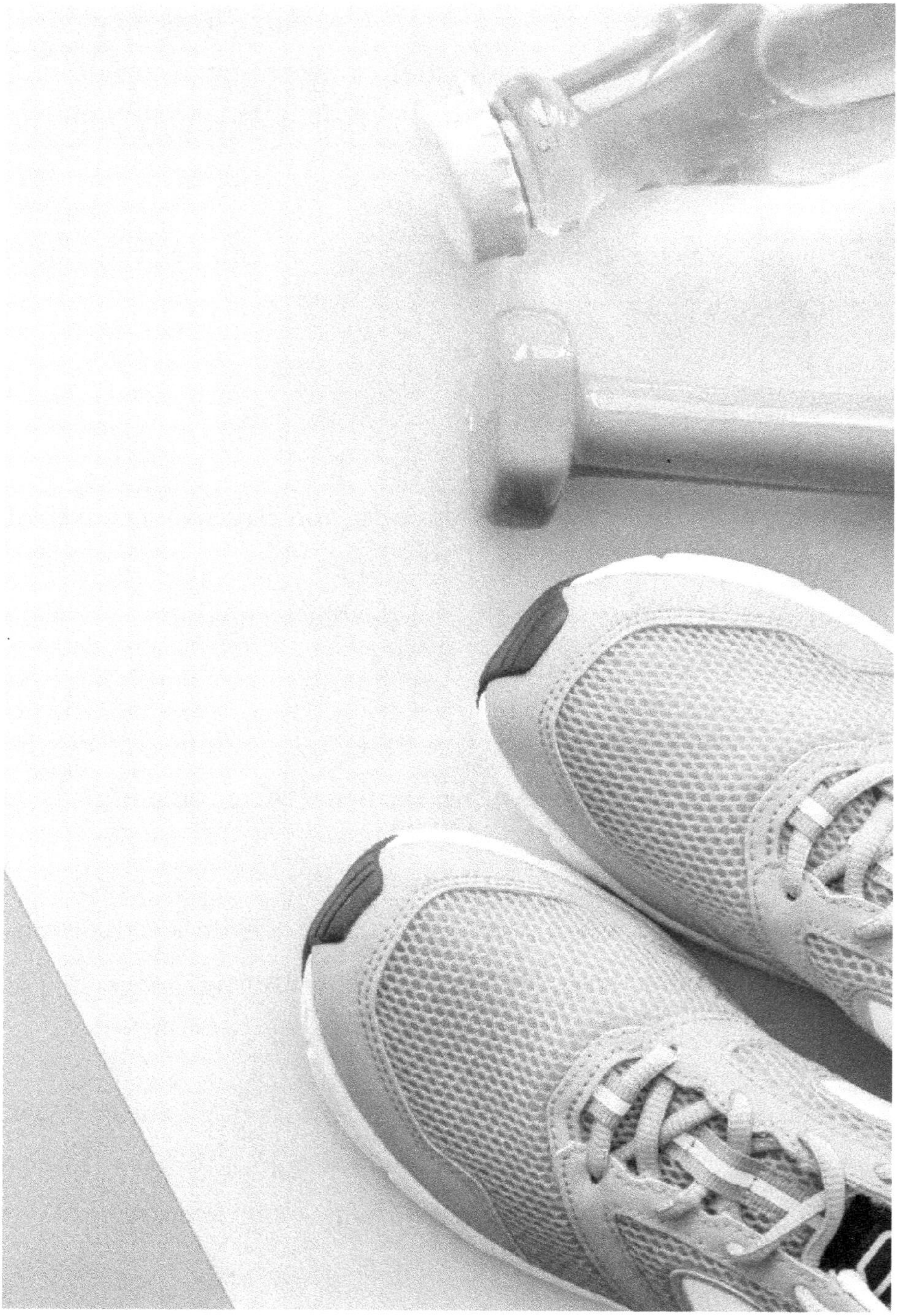

Chapter 5.
Meditation for Weight Loss

"The world we've created may be a product of our thinking. It can't be distorted without altering our thinking." – Einstein

This wonderful quote from Einstein clearly expresses the fundamentals of the Law of Attraction. It can be easily paraphrased and applied to the process of weight loss. For example, the body you have created is a product of your thinking. It CAN be changed by changing your thinking. So how do you change your thinking?

If you've been unhappy about your weight for many years, you may find it difficult to change your thinking. You may find it difficult to avoid thinking negatively about a few subjects with this much charge thereon.

The following Easy Weight Loss Meditation may be a powerful aid to extend your ability to vary your thoughts about your body from what you are doing not want to what you do want. This Easy Weight Loss Meditation is obtainable to support you in changing your brooding about your body so you'll see some real results NOW.

As you read the subsequent words, allow yourself to FEEL THIN. Allow yourself to sink deeply into feelings of living in your ideal body, and you'll easily and naturally change your brooding about your body. As you enjoy a relaxing journey to your inner world, you will be guided to IMAGINE YOURSELF THIN easily.

The Link between Meditation and Weight Loss

Some people have long thought that there is a link between meditation and long-term weight loss. When you meditate, you calm your body and concentrate on your breathing, which brings in oxygen, which in turn helps your body rejuvenated itself.

Doctors have disagreed on the role that meditation plays on weight loss. Some believe in the holistic medication route, while others believe only in science. Holistic medications include herbs, acupuncture, and meditation and relaxation techniques to help cleanse the toxins that may be harmful to your body and may hamper your weight loss goal.

Meditation can also help you maintain a healthy weight once you've reached your goal weight. Meditation will help you see the ideal weight you want to be and how you can maintain that ideal weight by visualizing a healthy you, warding off the bad foods, and other temptations.

On the other hand, meditation is not the only way to lose weight; it is a way to calm your mind and spirit while helping to cleanse your body through natural holistic foods.

This is a centuries-old tradition that may work for you if you give it a little time and concentrate and believe that it will work.

Holistic health addresses the mind and body, the spirit, and emotions - the entire body. Holistic health foods help cleanse your body of toxins such as metals from your drinking water and many unhealthy germs that you may come in contact with during daily life.

These holistic foods and natural grains help cleanse your body and rid you of toxins so that you feel better, healthier, and have more energy to do the things you want to do.

Eating holistic foods is a lifestyle change, not a diet, because diets don't work. You must change the way you think and feel about foods before you can begin to lose weight. You must think about what you're putting into your body in terms of food, is it a healthy food? Or is it bad food? Will this food help to promote a healthy body, which is what I want? Or will this food only satisfy my craving at this moment?

These are all things you need to ask yourself before allowing yourself to eat whatever it is you're about to eat. You can do this repeatedly, or you can change your lifestyle and begin with natural, holistic, and healthy foods and not worry about all the questions.

The combination of healthy foods and meditation can get you started to help the mind, body, and spirit. You will have boundless energy; you will feel so much better than you did before, and you will find that you will be able to do the things that you once were unable to do.

If you keep doing the meditation and eating a healthy diet, you will maintain a healthy weight. But remember it starts with a lifestyle change, not just adding good foods and a walk around the block, that's a diet and diet don't work but lifestyle changes do. You have to understand that you need to change your life to save your life from diabetes, obesity, heart disease, and a whole host of other complications due to being overweight.

Does Meditation For Weight Loss Work?

In case you're attempting to shed pounds, you presumably recognize what a disappointing encounter it tends to be. It's very simple to become involved with the yo-yo pattern of losing and afterward recovering. Tragically, numerous individuals never figure out how to break liberated from this.

In any case, some are understanding that there's a whole other world to getting in shape than simply controlling food admission and movement levels, and are finding that contemplation can be a significant expansion to any weight reduction system. In this part, we'll take a look at reflection for weight reduction in extra detail.

Why Meditate?

Reflection has been broadly concentrated as of late. Science is coming to acknowledge what smarter societies around the globe have referred to for a considerable length of time - that reflects the same number of advantages for physical and emotional wellness.

Meditation can assist in monitoring,focusing on levels, which can, thusly, make you more averse to build up an assortment of ailments, from coronary illness to stroke.

Meditation additionally includes a useful impact on your mental state. Meditators are often more joyful and more satisfied than individuals who don't meditate.

Reflection can be as basic as sitting or resting in an agreeable spot and simply putting your attention on your relaxing for a few minutes every day.

It doesn't need to be difficult work, and actually, the less complex your reflection system, the better, from multiple points of view.

Using meditation to assist you in weight loss

Meditation is often a valuable weight loss aid for various reasons. We've already noted that meditation features a very calming effect on the mind. This makes it invaluable to anybody who's susceptible to overeating as a response to anxiety or stress - as very many overweight people are. By meditating regularly, you've got an efficient tool that helps to stay your stress levels in check without turning to food. Once this tendency to eat for emotional reasons has been brought in to see, weight loss becomes much easier.

Another way that meditation can assist you in reducing is that it makes visualization simpler. Visualizing involves creating an image of whatever it's you would like to realize. In this case, you would possibly imagine yourself being as slim, healthy, and energetic as you would like to be, and maybe enjoying eating healthy food and exercise also. (Despite the name, it isn't necessary to make a visible image of your required state to see - instead, you'll specialize in how it'll feel to succeed in your goal or to listen to positive comments from others. do not be postpone the notion of visualizing if you're one among the various people that find it difficult to make mental pictures, as this is not necessary.)

With meditation, visualization is simpler, because meditation makes it easier to deeply relax and quieten your mind, which successively helps you to remain focused on your visualization and to implant it more firmly into your subconscious. With regular practice, such a weight loss visualization are often a really powerful way of adjusting your self-image, which successively helps to eliminate self-sabotaging behaviors, causes you to feel good about yourself, and makes it easier to accept a healthy way of life without having to force yourself to try to do so by means of willpower alone.

The only trouble with using meditation for weight loss is that a lot of people find it difficult to meditate, just because they are not won't keep their minds in check. Fortunately, however, an answer is out there in brainwave entrainment technologies like isochronic tones or binaural beats.

What Is Brainwave Entrainment?

Simply put, brainwave entrainment involves exposure to a repetitive stimulus like the sound of specific frequencies. The brain features a natural tendency to match its brainwave output to the frequencies of sounds it's hearing.

This is often useful because once you enter a deeply relaxed state, your brain activity slows down naturally.

If you discover this level of relaxation hard to realize on your own, taking note of a brainwave entrainment recording can lead your brain down into the specified state.

In this way, using binaural beats or other methods makes meditation much easier and more available to those that do not have years of experience with it already. you'll also begin to experience the advantages of meditation more quickly and simply than you'd use traditional techniques, which can take an extended time to master.

So, if you're uninterested in struggling to reduce, and constantly battling cravings using willpower alone, you ought to consider making meditation a part of your weight loss efforts. It does work, because the entire fat loss process becomes much easier once you've your mind on your side, and by means of brainwave entrainment makes it easier.

How Can Meditation Help Weight Loss?

Astonishing because it could also be, meditation for weight loss - particularly 'mindful meditation' - is increasingly getting used by people eager to control food cravings and manage to overeat. Mindful meditation also can be wont to control stress, thereby preventing 'comfort eating' borne out of that stress.

As we cultivate more mindful, we turn out to be more conscious of our cravings and may learn to concentrate on the emotions underlying them - i.e., we will make a more informed choice before simply reaching for that naughty chocolate bar! If you practice mindful eating a day, then in time, you'll learn to enjoy your food more. You'll even be better ready to recognize once you are full - meaning you'll naturally start consuming fewer calories.

Regular performance of mindful meditation has been revealed to reduce the strain hormone cortisol. This is often good news because high cortisol levels can cause pre-diabetes and central obesity (which is related to heart disease). Plus, cortisol starts a cascade in our brains, resulting in a much bigger appetite and large cravings.

What's Being Mindful?

During 'mindful' meditation, your goal is to remain 'mindful' or 'aware constantly'. When thoughts sneak into your mind, you can first recognize them, and secondly, 'let them go.' When you practice meditation for weight loss, lots of mental 'junk' and 'clutter' is bound to come up.

This incorporates negative self-perceptions and wants for food where they exist.

The uplifting news is, the more you practice meditation methods the easier it becomes to put these thoughts and their accompanying emotions quickly and directly into your 'mental recycling bin.' Also, 'mindful' eating - that's the process of eating slowly and silently whilst concentrating on the food only during your mealtimes - can help you become more in tune with your body's natural cues. You become improved able to stop eating before you are stuffed full.

Meditation for Weight Loss - Tips for Weight Loss

1. Don't Multi-Task

Experts say our biggest enemy in weight control is multi-tasking. Think over it... when was the last time you ate your lunch in complete peace and quiet, without flicking through your phone, tapping away on your computer, or chatting with work colleagues? When you practice mindful meditation for weight loss, it's important to concentrate on the food and the food alone. Why?

A recent study published in the journal 'Psychological Science' found that people who watched television during dinner were more likely to overeat because they found the food bland.

2. Don't Speed Eat

According to a survey by a group called 'Conscious Foods,' the average person gulps up all their food for the day - i.e., three meals' worth - in a total of just 23 minutes.

Eating too fast has been linked to weight gain and harmful diseases, including type 2 diabetes.

Try not to eat as though you are in a race. Contemplate and savor every bite of every meal - ensuring you taste it! You should ideally spend at least 20 minutes on each meal.

3. Consider Your Environment

When you practice meditation for weight loss, avoid bright lights and fast-paced music.

It can encourage you to eat faster and thus consume more calories.

It would help if you also ate from a smaller plate, to promote your mind to be satisfied with a smaller serving. Consider placing your knife and fork down between every bite.

4. Try 5 Breaths

It is essential to set the scene before you begin to eat. Taking five deep breaths before a meal relaxes the body and clears the emotional palate.

You can also try this halfway through a meal.

Top Benefits Of Meditation For Weight Loss

Can I lose weight with meditation? It is a multi-billion dollar industry that primarily and banks on you consuming more foods to keep the weight-loss craze alive. Ironic! Can meditation help you lose weight? The benefits of meditation have been brilliantly documented for the mind body-positive results. Here is my take.

The day-to-day grind allows us to hold all the tension and stress in our bodies, whether we realize it. Getting to work, dealing with difficult people, paying the bills, all the commitments and obligations are all vessels of some concerns that lead to clogging, and blocking our energy. We can hold all this nervous energy in our bodies, our organs, and our every cell level.

Meditation can ease, open blockages, and provide an optimum environment for healing and wellness evolution of the body. If the organs can relax just enough to allow more energy to move and resolve the negative blockages on its own, then everything we consume in our body flows better.

Top Benefits of Meditation for Weight Loss:

1. Get more energy.

Meditating three to five minutes a day will give your mind and body a chance to rest, relax, rejuvenate, and recharge your body down to every cell.

2. Feel Good.

The better you feel, the happier you will be, the easier it is to lose the pounds. If you're a stress eater, instead of grabbing a sweet cake, try meditating for a few minutes until the craving goes away. Try it!

3. Better focus.

The more you meditate, the better you will be able to focus. Meditating is also the practice of focusing on clear intentions. The better you can focus, the better you will be able to focus on achieving your weight goals.

4. Reduce Stress and Anxiety.

Some folks go to the gym to relieve stress, so can meditation. Even if you exorcize your body and you are still stressed out, the body will still be holding all that tension. If the mind is holding you back, so will your body. Why not do both.

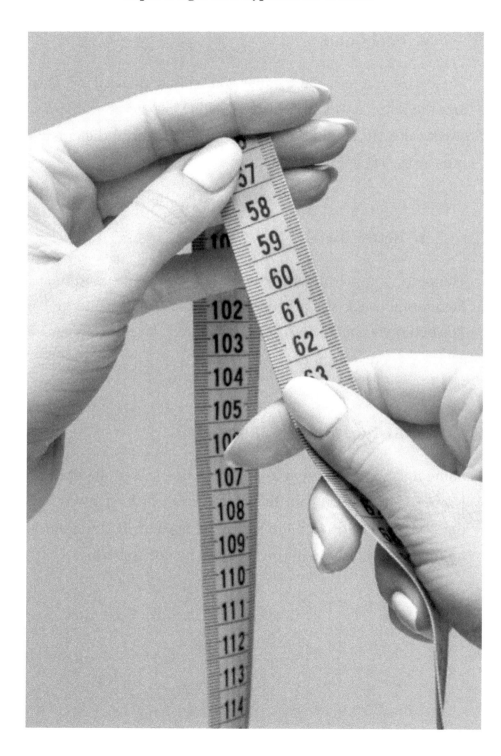

Chapter 6.
Daily weight loss meditation

W hether it is to be healthy, everybody wants to lose weight and look fit. Unhealthy lifestyles often include tons of junk and oily food, alongside little or no or no exercise.

Sitting in your work seat can make all the fats gather in the lower some portion of your body, in this manner focusing on your thighs and hips. Fat in the hips and thighs is known as cellulite.Cellulite is firm and may prove pretty difficult to urge obviate.

Here are some recommendations on the way to lessen hip fat:

1.   Drink Water

This arrangement appears as though it won't have a great deal of effects; however it assumes a huge job in controlling your weight. There is a motivation behind why all wellbeing specialists underline its criticalness. Water cleans your framework and discharges undesirable poisons off the body.

It likewise helps digestion, subsequently expanding the pace of your weight reduction venture. It's prescribed to devour in any event 8-9 glasses each day for one to remain sound. You can likewise crush some juice in your water for included advantages.

2.   Reduce Sugars

Cut down on your utilization of sugar as chocolates and desserts. Sugar is an immediate type of fat and the essential explanation that causes fat hips. Supplant your sweet longings with organic products. Sodas and circulated air through beverages are the same amount of stacked with colossal measures of undesirable sugar.

3.   Exercise

One of the basic hints to reduce weight is workout. Normal exercises are important for cutting back fat and controlling excess gathering. Activities that increase the cells in your body are becoming increasingly serious and require more exertion. You ought to preferably exercise for at any rate 30 minutes consistently.

Your day by day exercise must subsume practices like squats, sit-ups, crunches, jumps, and hip raises in different checks and requests. These activities focus principally on the correct forming of your hips and thighs. They are profoundly serious and will be joined with cardio consistently. You can likewise secure blood flow and lift digestion, successfully consuming fats by lively strolling, running, and running.

4.   Control Calories

Avoid garbage and prepared food, much the same as the plague! They have next to zero to no dietary benefit and contribute literally nothing towards weight reduction. They are the additional calories that hinder your way to sound objectives. Ensure that your dinners consistently incorporate green, verdant vegetables to ad-lib your nourishing admission.

It should likewise contain proteins and nutrients in a greater number of amounts than starches and sugars. Forestall eating as much as possible. Try not to eat constantly; rather, eat satisfying dinners to keep visit hunger under control.

5.   Yoga

Yoga and meditation help in quieting your nerves and balancing out pulse. In case you don't have enough time to go through a yoga schedule a day, you should at least carry out a breathing activity for a few minutes toward the beginning of the day. A casual body is certainly a solid body.

Wellness will be a long excursion loaded with a sound eating regimen and exercise schedule. Continually keeping a mind what you eat and keep up a legitimate exercise system is the most ideal approach to keep up solid and recommendable weight. Hips might be an extreme territory to trim.

Still, with the correct mindset, dedication & determination, a slimmer waist is all yours. Plan your fitness journey accordingly and the go-ahead to that wedding function or a vacation with a fitter version of you!

Meditation for Weight Loss: The Right Routine

Meditation will help you lose weight if you rely on appropriate practices. The idea is to find the right frame of mind to enjoy your meals in the best possible conditions. And therefore lose the excess weight due to your negative emotions.

The essential rule here is to live in the present moment. These few questions will guide you in the right direction.

Before the meal

- Identify your hunger: go to the table because you are hungry? By habit? Because you have to eat? To spend social time with family, friends,…?

- Is your hunger devouring, reasonable, or downright non-existent?

- Do you want, sweet? Salty? Dry (nuts, almonds, etc.)? Wet (mash, compote...)? Cold? Hot? ...

• Identify your emotions: how do you feel? Hurry)? Stressed)? Calm? Relaxed? In a bad mood?

During the meal

Avoid distractions. Cut TV, mobile, social networks...;

Concentrate on your plate and its content;

Admire the color, the shape of the food, its arrangement on your plate;

Appreciate their flavors, their smells, and their texture;

Chew carefully to capture the slightest taste: salty, sweet, spicy, etc.

After lunch

Identify your emotions: have you eaten enough? Not enough? Are you relaxed? Are you satisfied?

At least at the beginning, try to submit yourself to these questions. Afterward, your brain will take care of itself to send you a precise massage on your state of being.

All of this will directly affect the quality of your life in general and your health in particular. Not to mention that in the meantime, you will get closer to your goal of losing weight, without any special diet.

How every day Meditation Can Help You Lose Weight

You've presumably taken a stab at everything to shed off those bothersome pounds, from confining your calories to heightening your exercise schedule.While these efforts could be helping you shed a pound or two every few weeks, there's something which will offer you that extra boost of awareness.

This cost-free, natural, simple strategy is often very effective in helping you reduce, while additionally reducing pressure and nervousness. The examination encompassing careful contemplation rehearses recommends that reflection is firmly connected to weight reduction.

The ideas of care and reflection can't just lower your feelings of anxiety and lift mindfulness. Having a mindful brain can keep you from voraciously consuming food and passionate eating.

Consequently, reflection for weight reduction can be a sound and compelling approach to get in shape and eat better.

About Meditation

Basically, reflection is the demonstration of concentrating the eye on getting increasingly careful.

As per the American Meditation Society, during reflection, an individual's consideration essentially streams inwards as opposed to drawing in inside the external universe of action.

The practice involves clearing the mind to return to a state of calm emotions and straightforward thinking.

Some people practice meditation for less than five minutes each day. However, experts are suggesting trying to work that up to about 20 minutes a day.

For those who're simply beginning, consider taking five minutes soon after you wake up to clear your brain before continuing ahead with your day.

If you don't mind close your eyes and spotlight on your breathing example without attempting to transform it. On the off chance that your brain meanders, which is very regular when beginning, direct it back to your relaxing.

How To make sure that Daily Meditation for Weight Loss Works for You

❖ **Choose the proper practice.**

There are several different meditation styles that you simply can accompany, though all of them follow an identical basic technique of calming the mind and taking a while to breathe and becoming conscious of this moment. It knows to try a variety of methods that sound interesting to you to seek out which of them work best.

❖ **Reflect on Aromatherapy**

This has also been confirmed to be effective in calming the body, which is useful when meditating. You'll generally use aromatherapy for meditation in two alternative ways. The primary is diffusing the oil into the air.

This can help promote relaxation, stimulate the senses, and make an ambient space where you'll really focus. Alternatively, try using essential oils during a personal aromatherapy diffuser like Zen, Vibrant, Active, or Healthy MONQ. Gently breathe MONQ into your mouth then out through your nose. MONQ shouldn't be inhaled into the lungs.

Additionally, essential oils are often applied topically to the skin after dilution with a carrier oil.

❖ Hone the Practice

Some books teach you ways to meditate. Those that are new to the concept of meditation can particularly enjoy these. If you'd have an interest in undertaking meditation during a guided group setting, consider trying out your local meditation center. Most towns and concrete centers have facilities or schools where mediators of varied levels close to practice.

Mindfulness and Meditation in Action

Meditation and mindfulness are recognized to improve psychological wellbeing. Mindfulness has been revealed to lessen emotional eating, binge eating, and usually enhancing weight loss.

Chronic stress is related to a greater concentration of fats within the abdomen, especially through the overproduction of the strain hormone cortisol, which is additionally linked to higher mortality. Because of this connection, an investigation from the University of California at San Francisco concentrated on distinguishing in the case of bringing down feelings of anxiety through contemplation can really help bring down the centralization of belly fat.

The study was published in 2011 within the Journal of Obesity and researched a gaggle of 47 obese or overweight female participants (with a mean of 31.2 bodies mass index), giving half them a series of classes about mindfulness meditation techniques.

The classes included instructing them while in transit to focus on impressions of food desires, hunger, recognize passionate eating triggers, learn self-acknowledgment, and become aware of negative feelings. The guided reflections were given to present new careful eating aptitudes, such as giving close consideration to the flavor of food, likewise as eating more gradually than expected.

All in all, the investigation group got nine classes, each enduring over two hours, nearby a quiet retreat day where they were urged to rehearse their new careful eating and reflection abilities. They were additionally urged to utilize the careful aptitudes once they got a range in assignments of up to half-hour out of every day during or before suppers, six days consistently, and to sign in their contemplation movement.

Both the control groups and, therefore, the study group received also received two-hour nutrition and exercise information sessions. At the top of the research period, all of the participants were measured for his or her distribution and amount of abdominal fat, alongside their cortisol level.

Two key results of the investigation were assessed: regardless of whether the strain decrease and careful eating program diminished passionate eating and whether it influenced the amount of paunch fat in members. All in all, the investigation found these rehearsed diminished enthusiastic eating, decreased feelings of anxiety, expanded consciousness of their real sensations, and diminished food desires.

Furthermore, blood cortisol levels were lower inside the treatment group contrasted with the benchmark group.

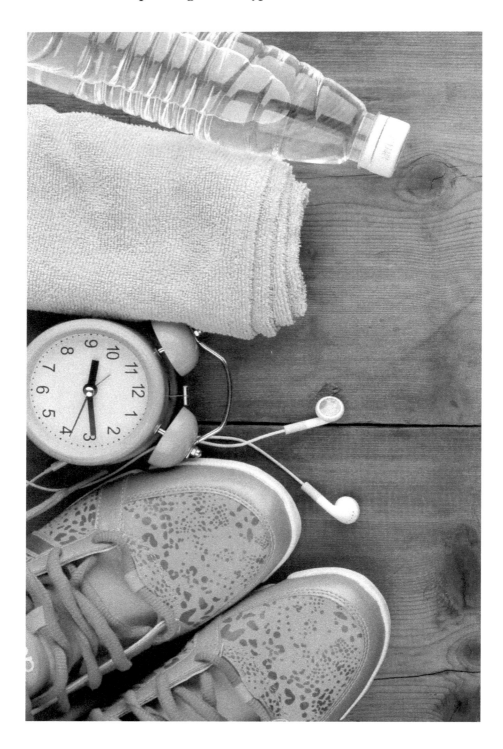

Conclusion

H ypnosis is a dream state in which you are focused on a particular area. It is very similar to REM (rapid eye movement) sleep, which is an important part of rejuvenating your body.

Most people don't have problems going to sleep at night. Once you realize that hypnosis is a slightly different form of essential sleep, you can relax and feel confident that you are not being controlled by someone else.

While hypnotized, you still can think logically. Other portions of your mind are just more open to change. You are in control at all times. The hypnotist is just there to help you. A hypnotist must be flexible and adaptable to be effective. Each subject is different, so each hypnosis session must also be unique.

Hypnosis is not a form of entertainment. It is a life-changing process that works with most people. Heroin addicts can get off of the drugs and stay off of them. Hypnosis for weight loss will keep the pounds off for good.

This technique can change your life for the better in so many ways. If you have an area that you are struggling with and conquer it with the help of hypnosis, you will also gain confidence in other areas. Your whole life can change as a result of successful hypnosis.

Hypnosis is a great learning tool that can be used by almost any human being. A slightly different form of hypnosis is used every time you focus on something and give it your undivided attention. You need to be comfortable with hypnosis for it to work.

Think of it as your friend. Hypnosis is a natural process that many use daily. You often don't even know they are doing so. Anyone can learn and be helpedby this technique, and you do not have to worry about side effects. There are none with this behavior modification method.

CPSIA information can be obtained
at www.ICGtesting.com
Printed in the USA
BVHW010853250621
610445BV00002B/103